Mary. I. Thomson
59 URQUHART ROAD
ABERDEEN
AB2 1NA.

NEUROLOGY

MODERN NURSING SERIES

General Editors
A. J. HARDING RAINS M.S., F.R.C.S.
MISS VALERIE HUNT S.R.N., S.C.M., O.N.D., R.N.T.

A SELECTION OF TITLES AVAILABLE AS PAPERBACKS

Textbook of Medicine
with relevance to physiology and anatomy
R. J. HARRISON ch.B., M.D.

Psychology and Psychiatry for Nurses
PETER J. DALLY M.B., F.R.C.P., D.P.M.
HEATHER HARRINGTON S.R.N., R.M.N.

Revision Notes on Psychiatry
K. T. KOSHY S.R.N., R.M.N., B.T.A., R.N.T., A.R.I.P.H.H., M.R.S.H.

Venereology for Nurses
R. D. CATTERALL F.R.C.P.(Edin.)

Pathology
C. P. MAYERS M.R.C.Path.

Communicable Diseases
W. PARRY M.D., D.P.H., D.T.M.&H.

Emergency and Acute Care
A. J. HARDING RAINS M.S., F.R.C.S.
KEITH W. REYNOLDS M.S., F.R.C.S.
VALERIE HUNT S.R.N., S.C.M., O.N.D., R.N.T.

Principles of Intensive Care
E. R. J. EMERY M.B., ch.B., F.F.A., D.A.
A. K. YATES M.B., ch.B., F.R.C.S.
P. J. MOORHEAD M.D., ch.B., M.R.C.P.

The Older Patient
a textbook of geriatrics
R. E. IRVINE M.A., M.D., F.R.C.P.
M. K. BAGNALL A.I.M.S.W.
B. J. SMITH S.R.N., R.F.N.

Ear, Nose and Throat Surgery and Nursing
R. PRACY M.B., B.S., F.R.C.S.
J. SIEGLER D.L.O., F.R.C.S.
P. M. STELL ch.M., F.R.C.S., A.I.L.
J. ROGERS M.A., F.R.C.S.

NEUROLOGY

EDWIN R. BICKERSTAFF

M.D., F.R.C.P.

Senior Consultant Neurologist, The Midland Centre for Neurosurgery and Neurology, Smethwick, West Midlands;
Honorary Consultant in Neurology, Birmingham Teaching Hospitals;
Senior Clinical Lecturer and Tutor in Neurology, and Postgraduate Clinical Tutor, University of Birmingham

Chapters 18 and 19 on Operative Neurosurgery by

PETER H. SCHURR

M.A., M.B., B.Chir., F.R.C.S.

Director, the Neurosurgical Unit of Guy's, Maudsley, and King's College Hospitals, London;
Sub-Dean of Postgraduate Studies, Guy's Hospital Medical School

HODDER AND STOUGHTON

LONDON SYDNEY AUCKLAND TORONTO

British Library Cataloguing in Publication Data
Bickerstaff, Edwin Robert
Neurology—3rd ed.
—(Modern nursing series).
1. Nervous system—Diseases
2. Neurological nursing
I. Title II. Schurr, Peter Howel III.
Series 616.8'02'4613 RC346

ISBN 0-340-23166-1
ISBN 0-340-23167-x Pbk

ISBN 0 340 23166 1 Boards
ISBN 0 340 23167 x Unibook

First printed 1965
Reprinted 1968, 1969, 1970
Second edition 1971
Reprinted 1973, 1974, 1975, 1977
Third edition 1978

Swedish edition published by Natur och Kultur, Stockholm
Italian edition published by Il Pensiero Scientifico, Rome

Printed in Great Britain for
Hodder and Stoughton Educational,
a division of Hodder and Stoughton Ltd.,
Mill Road, Dunton Green, Sevenoaks, Kent by
Richard Clay (The Chaucer Press), Ltd.,
Bungay, Suffolk.

EDITORS' FOREWORD

The scope of this series has increased since it was first established, and it now serves a wide range of medical, nursing and ancillary professions, in line with the present trend towards the belief that all who care for patients in a clinical context have an increasing amount in common.

The texts are carefully prepared and organized so that they may be readily kept up to date as the rapid developments of medical science demand. The series already includes many popular books on various aspects of medical and nursing care, and reflects the increased emphasis on community care.

The increasing specialization in the medical profession is fully appreciated and the books are often written by Physicians or Surgeons in conjunction with specialist nurses. For this reason, they will not only cover the syllabus of training of the General Nursing Council, but will be designed to meet the needs of those undertaking training controlled by the Joint Board of Clinical Studies set up in 1970.

PREFACE TO FIRST EDITION

Glancing along the crowded shelves labelled 'Books for Nurses' in libraries and bookshops, one is struck by the absence of text books devoted to diseases of the nervous system. Each book on general medicine, of course, has its section on neurology which is necessarily limited in its scope owing to lack of space. There are some excellent books on the bedside nursing of neurological and neurosurgical cases, but these say little about the nature of the diseases under treatment, their origin or their outlook. It is with these aspects of organic nervous disease that I have attempted to deal. It is important for the nurse to know about them, for these are cases specially needful of her care, and they are not just to be found segregated in special units, but abound in every general medical ward. I hope, therefore, that both the trainee and the postgraduate will find here the information that they need presented in a manner which they can understand and absorb, and which will interest them in this all-important branch of medicine.

A book is always the result of team work. I am particularly grateful to Professor A. J. Harding Rains, General Editor of this series, and Mr. John Maitland, of the English Universities Press, who first stimulated me into writing this book, and to Mr. Brian Steven and Mr. David Zwartz, who were so helpful during its production. Finally, my wife, herself an S.R.N. patiently typed and retyped the various versions of the manuscript, and her criticisms and advice have been invaluable in assessing what in particular a nurse wants to know, and how best to describe it to her.

PREFACE TO SECOND EDITION

It had always been my impression that nurses, physiotherapists, radiographers, electroencephalographers and laboratory technicians wanted a small book which explained in as straightforward a manner as possible the diseases of the nervous system they were called upon to treat or investigate, and the fact that within five years three reprints of the first edition have been required has rather confirmed this. However, there have been several changes in thought in the neurological field in this time, and this new edition gives me the opportunity to revise the whole book, rewrite several chapters, correct omissions, and clarify still further phrases or explanations which some readers found difficult or puzzling. The book's aim remains the same—to help the nurse and other hospital ancillary staff to know what the doctors mean when they are talking about their patients, the diseases they suffer from, and the investigations they are undertaking. It has grown a little, for neurology is constantly advancing, but I hope this adds to rather than detracts from its usefulness.

EDWIN R. BICKERSTAFF

The Midland Centre for Neurosurgery and Neurology

PREFACE TO THIRD EDITION

It is not until one starts preparing a new edition of a book such as this that one realises how considerable have been the advances in the understanding, investigation, and treatment of certain diseases of the nervous system in the past few years. During several reprints of the second edition brief reference has been possible to some of these, but the time has now come to revise the whole book, particularly in respect of the sections on cerebrovascular disease, encephalitis, syringomyelia, the treatment of Parkinsonism and epilepsy, and methods of neuroradiological investigation.

The neurologist and the neurosurgeon have come to work even more closely together and it is with great pleasure that I have been able to include two chapters on the principles of operative neurosurgery by Mr. Peter Schurr.

This book has become widely used as an elementary textbook for undergraduate medical students in editions translated into Swedish and Italian, and indeed is recommended as such in some parts of this country. Conscious of this I have tried to include some facets of the subject which the most junior students may find rather perplexing in their usual textbooks. However, the book retains its main and original purpose, which is to help the nurse, trained or in training, to know what the doctors mean when they talk about certain diseases, why they choose to carry out investigations in some but not all patients, and what are the reasons for the choice of particular forms of treatment. It is not, and never has been, a book on the techniques of nursing care for these can only be learnt at the bedside. But how much more interesting these techniques become when the nurse can understand why the team of which she or he is so important a member is taking a particular line of action.

As a gesture to conformity, and with admitted reluctance, I have given readings in the appendices in S.I. units as well as in their better-known values, in the hope that youth can assimilate what some of us find indigestible.

EDWIN R. BICKERSTAFF

The Midland Centre for Neurosurgery and Neurology

CONTENTS

1 *NEUROLOGY, NEUROLOGISTS AND NEUROLOGICAL NURSING*

The increasing popularity of books, films, and television plays about doctors and nurses might have been expected to clarify for the public what a neurologist is and what a neurologist does. Quite the reverse seems to be the case. There is still complete confusion in people's minds between neurology and psychiatry, and between neurologists and psychiatrists.

One can hardly blame the layman, for writers and producers frequently show how much they share this confusion, but remarks such as 'another day like this and I shall have to come and see *you*' are frequently made to the neurologist by those who should know better—nurses, physiotherapists, and, regrettably, sometimes even doctors.

Neurology is the study of the nervous system and of the diseases and disorders which affect it. By the nervous system is meant the brain, spinal cord, and peripheral nerves—definite structures which can be seen, felt, X-rayed, operated on, and looked at under a microscope.

Unfortunately the terms 'nervous', 'nervy', and 'the nerves' are often used to describe purely emotional states which are quite unrelated to disease of the central nervous system. In some countries neurology and psychiatry are both practised by the same people, working under the name neuropsychiatrists, and, in fact, the two branches of medicine do at times overlap, for disease of certain parts of the brain can cause profound mental disturbance. It is hardly surprising, therefore, that many think they should see a neurologist when their 'nerves' are in bad shape.

Confusion of this sort would not matter very much if sometimes it did not have rather serious results. Patients may resist being referred to or admitted to a neurological unit because they are convinced it is a 'cover-up' name for a mental hospital, and an early and treatable stage of a disease may be missed. Nurses also, wishing to nurse organic disease, are often reluctant to work in neurological units because they have gained the same impression.

Sadly, however, reluctance to take up neurological nursing has another equally incorrect origin. The idea is widely held that all neurological diseases are chronic, crippling, untreatable, and as depressing to nurse as they are to endure. Nothing could be further from the truth. Such diseases exist, of course, as in all other branches of medicine, but the advances of the last twenty years have been dramatic, and as most of the patients in an active neurological unit are mentally normal, feel physically well, and are in the younger two-thirds of life, they form a group who are most pleasant to deal with, and most rewarding to nurse.

False ideas about neurosurgery are even worse, for they have spread even amongst the medical profession. The neurosurgeon is thought to spend his time carrying out leucotomies on mental patients, or being called in as a last resort for hopeless head injuries, or inoperable tumours. In fact, a neurosurgeon in an active department concentrates on the vast number of patients with eminently treatable conditions, who are operated on, recover rapidly, and return home to active life. There are, of course, bad cases, as in all other branches, and as these often return from a neurosurgical unit to a general ward or hospital, and there deteriorate and die, they are remembered as 'typical neurosurgical cases'. When, however, general physicians, surgeons, or nurses visit a neurosurgical unit, they are invariably astonished to see how small a proportion of the work is made up of this type of case.

To the nurse the process of diagnosis in neurological disease is itself fascinating. It is easy to see the physical signs being demonstrated; the investigations, particularly the X-ray studies, generally give clear-cut results which everyone can see, so that the nurse need not be just a patient bystander; each case is like a detective story in which the nurses themselves, by using their powers of observation, often furnish the vital clues which solve the diagnostic problem.

Neurology, however, abounds with long words. These may slip off the experienced physician's tongue before he realises that his audience is still thinking about the last one. A chapter is therefore devoted to the meaning of the words which are most commonly used. This is followed by those bare essentials of the anatomy and function of the nervous system which have to be appreciated so that the way in which the various diseases affect the body may be understood. In the rest of the book the nurse will find an outline of all the neurological diseases which occur with any frequency, and as simple an explanation as possible of their causes, if these are known, so that when she hears a particular diagnosis being discussed she will know what it means, how it may have developed, and what is likely to happen to the patient.

Knowledge of this sort not only makes it easier to talk to the patients and their relatives, but greatly increases the interest of each problem in what is one of the most interesting branches of medicine.

2 *THE LANGUAGE OF NEUROLOGY*

This chapter gives the meaning of words commonly used in neurology, which are either special to the subject, or have a special meaning when applied to neurological cases. Terms familiar from general medicine are not included, nor are the names of diseases, for these are defined in the chapters that follow.

A- (or An-). Absence of—or inability to—.
Abdominal reflexes. Abdominal muscle contractions on stroking the skin.
Air-encephalography (pneumoencephalography). X-raying the ventricles and subarachnoid spaces after introduction of air by lumbar or cisternal puncture.
Air-myelography. X-raying the spinal canal after injection of air.
Akinesia. Inability to start a movement; slowness in movement.
Amnesia. Loss of memory.
Anaesthesia. Inability to feel touch.
Analgesia. Inability to feel pain.
Anarthria. Inability to pronounce words.
Anastomosis. Network of vessels (replacing one that is blocked).
Aneurysm. A weak bulge in an arterial wall.
Angioma. A collection of abnormal arteries, capillaries, and veins.
Anosmia. Loss of sense of smell.
Anterior horns. Part of spinal grey matter containing motor nerve cells.
Anticonvulsants. Drugs used to control epileptic fits.
Aphasia. Inability to speak.
Aphonia. Inability to make sounds.
Arachnoid mater. The web-like middle layer of the meninges.
Argyll Robertson pupil. An irregular pupil reacting to convergence but not to light.
Arteriography (-gram). X-raying blood-vessels after injecting an artery with opaque dye.
Astereognosis. Inability to recognise objects by size and shape.
Ataxia. Unsteadiness.
Athetosis. Slow writhing involuntary movements.
Aura. Warning symptoms (of an attack of epilepsy or migraine).
Axon. The longest process of a nerve cell.

Babinski reflex (sign). Extension of the great toe on scratching the sole.
Bitemporal hemianopia. Loss of the outer halves of both fields of vision.
Brown-Séquard syndrome. Signs produced by damage to one half of the cord.
Bruit (intracranial). A sound in time with the heart beat.
Bulbar. Concerning the medulla.
Burr-hole. A hole drilled in the skull.

Café-au-lait patches. Brown skin marks in neurofibromatosis.
Capsule. Fibrous barrier around a tumour or abscess.
Carpal Tunnel. Channel in wrist through which the median nerve passes.
C.A.T. Computerised axial tomography (E.M.I. scanner).
Cauda equina. The nerve fibres lying below the spinal cord.
Cephalgia. Headache.
Cerebellar. Concerning the cerebellum.
Cerebral. Concerning the brain.
Charcot's joints. Painless disorganised joints in tabes.
Chiasma (-al). The X-like crossing of the two optic nerves.
Chorea. Very rapid involuntary movements.
Choroid plexus. Tufts of vascular tissue in the ventricles forming the C.S.F.
Circle of Willis. The arteries at the base of the brain.
Cisterns. Collections of C.S.F. (e.g. cisterna magna).
Clonus (-ic). Rhythmical contractions of a spastic muscle on stretching.
Coma. Deep loss of consciousness.
Contrast media. Substances used to show up blood vessels or C.S.F. pathways on X-ray—'positive' if more opaque than bone and brain, 'negative' if less.
Co-ordination. Smooth and efficient movement.
Corneal reflex. Normal blinking on touching the cornea.
Cortex. The surface layer of the cerebral and cerebellar hemispheres.
Cranial nerves. 12 pairs arising from or running to the brain and brain stem.
C.S.F. The cerebro-spinal fluid, bathing brain and spinal cord.

Deficiency disease. One due to lack of a normal food substance.
Degeneration. Death of tissue, often of unknown cause.
Déjà-vu. A sense of familiarity.
Dementia. Deterioration of intellect.
Demyelinative. Due to loss of the myelin sheath.
Diabetes insipidus. Passage of large amounts of sugar-free urine.

Diplopia. Seeing double.

Disc (optic). The optic nerve leaving the eye, seen through an opthalmoscope.

Disc (intervertebral). The fibro-cartilaginous cushion between the vertebrae.

Discriminative sense. Ability to detect difference in size, shape, texture and number of stimuli.

Disorientation. Confusion as to time, place, person.

Dissociated sensory loss. Loss of pain sense with light touch preserved.

Dominant hemisphere. The cerebral hemisphere controlling speech.

Dorsiflexion. Bending backwards (usually wrist or ankle).

Drop attacks. Sudden falls without loss of consciousness.

Dura mater. The outer, toughest sheet of meninges.

Dys-. Difficulty in—.

Dysarthria. Difficulty in pronouncing words.

Dysgraphia. Difficulty in writing.

Dyslexia. Difficulty in reading.

Dysphasia. Difficulty in expressing thoughts in words.

Dystrophy. Degeneration with loss of function.

Echo-encephalography. Using ultra-sound to detect intracranial lesions.

Electrocorticography. Recording electrical activity direct from the cortex.

Electroencephalography (E.E.G.). Recording the electrical activity of the brain.

Electromyography (E.M.G.). Recording the electrical activity of muscle.

Electrophoresis. A method of separating the proteins in blood or C.S.F.

Encephalitis (plural, **encephalitides**). Inflammation of the brain.

Encephalopathy. A disorder of brain function.

Euphoria. A casual cheerfulness.

Extensor plantar response. The big toe goes up on scratching the sole.

Extracranial. Outside the skull.

Extradural. Between the dura and the skull.

Extrapyramidal. Motor fibres arising from cells other than the pyramidal cells (often basal ganglia).

Extrinsic. Outside and separate from nervous tissue.

Fasciculation. Flickering contractions of muscle fibres.

Flaccid. Limp; floppy; loss of tone.

Flexor plantar response. The normal downward movement of the big toe on scratching the foot.
Flexor spasm. Painful contractions of muscles in spastic limbs.
Focal. Arising from, or limited to, one part.
Focal epilepsy. A fit affecting one part of the body, arising from one point in the brain.
Foramen. An opening.
Fortification spectra. Zig-zag patterns seen in migraine.
Fossa. A compartment of the skull holding a part of the brain.
Functional. Due to a disturbance in the working, not the structure, of some part.

Gamma-camera. Apparatus for photographing uptake of radioisotopes in intracranial lesions (γ-scanning).
Ganglia. Collections of nerve cells.
Generalised fits. Convulsions affecting all parts of the body.
Girdle pains. Constricting pains around the trunk.
Glia. The supporting cells and fibres of the nervous system.
Glioblastoma. The most malignant glioma.
Glioma. Tumours growing from the supporting cells.
Gliosis. Overgrowth of glial fibres.
Glove and stocking anaesthesia. Impaired sensation over the periphery of all four limbs.
Grand mal. Epilepsy characterised by major fits.
Grey matter. Nervous tissue containing nerve cells.
Gyri. The folds of the cerebral cortex.

Hallucinations. Sensory impressions of something which is not there.
Hemianaesthesia. Loss of sensation down one side of the body.
Hemianopia. Loss of half the visual field.
Hemiplegia (-paresis). Paralysis (weakness) of one half of the body.
Heredo-familial. Passed both from generation to generation and to several members of one family.
Herpes simplex. The virus of 'cold sores'.
Herpes zoster. Shingles.
Hiatus. A large gap.
Homonymous. The same on both sides.
Hydrocephalus. Enlargement of the ventricles.
Hydrocephalus (low pressure). Ditto, when C.S.F. pressure is not high.
Hyper-. Increased.
Hypertrophy. Enlargement.
Hyperventilation. Excessively deep and fast breathing.
Hypo-. Decreased.

Hypoglycaemia. An abnormally low blood sugar.
Hypopituitarism. Loss of pituitary function.

Idiopathic. Of unknown cause.
Impulses. Electrical waves travelling along nerves.
Inborn. Part of an individual's make-up.
Infarct. A zone of tissue deprived of blood supply.
Intracranial. Inside the skull.
Intracranial hypertension. High pressure inside the skull (not high blood pressure).
Intrinsic. Inside the substance of the nervous system.
Involuntary movement. Muscular activity not under the patient's control.
Ischaemia. Shortage of blood supply.

Jacksonian fits. Convulsions starting at one point and spreading to involve wider areas.

Kernig's sign. Inability to straighten the knee with the hip flexed, in meningeal irritation.

Labyrinth. The semi-circular canals of the inner ear.
Lange curve. A test carried out by adding C.S.F. to colloidal gold solution.
Lasègue's sign. Limitation of straight leg raising.
Leucodystrophy. Degeneration of white matter.
Lightning pains. Needle-like pains in the limbs in tabes.
Lobe. A major division of the cerebral hemispheres or cerebellum.
Local; localise. One point affected; to determine the exact point affected.
Lower motor neurone. Cells and fibres of motor cranial and spinal nerves.

Medulla. The lowest part of the brain stem.
Meninges. The three membranes clothing the brain and cord and lining the skull and vertebral canal.
Meningioma. A benign tumour growing from the arachnoid.
Meningism. Signs of irritation of the meninges, not due to infection.
Meningitis. Inflammation of the meninges.
Meningocele. A bulge of the meninges through a breach in the bony coverings.
Meningo-encephalitis. Inflammation of both brain and meninges.
Meningomyelocele. A meningocele containing spinal cord tissue.
Mixed nerve. One containing motor and sensory fibres.
Monoplegia (-paresis). Paralysis of one limb.

Motor. Concerned with movement.
Multiple sclerosis. Disseminated sclerosis.
Myasthenia. Weakness of muscle.
Myelin. The white sheath to nerve fibres.
Myelitis. Inflammation of the spinal cord.
Myelography (myelogram). X-raying the vertebral canal by introducing opaque fluid into the C.S.F.
Myoclonus. Shock-like muscle contractions.
Myopathy. Degenerative disease of muscle (muscular dystrophy).
Myositis. Inflammation of muscle.
Myotonia. Contraction of muscle persisting after the need for it has passed.

Neck-stiffness, rigidity, retraction. Signs of irritation or infection of the meninges.
Nerve conduction time. Time taken for an electrical impulse to travel along an known length of nerve.
Neuralgia. Pain in the distribution of a nerve.
Neuritis. Inflammation of a nerve.
Neuromuscular junction. A point where a nerve fibre ends in a muscle.
Neurone. The nerve cell, its fibre and all its branches.
Neurosyphilis. Involvement of the nervous system in the later stages of syphilis.
Nucleus (-ei). A collection(s) of nerve cells.
Nystagmus. Rhythmical oscillation of the eyes.

Oculomotor. Concerned with eye movement.
Olfactory. Concerned with the sense of smell.
Oligophrenia. Mental retardation.
Ophthalmoplegia (-ic). Paralysis of eye movement.
Opisthotonos. Backward arching of the whole body.
Optic. Concerned with the eyes or visual pathways.
Organic. Due to structural disease.
Otorrhoea. Running from the ear.
Overflow incontinence. Constant dribbling due to over-distension of an insensitive bladder.

Panencephalitis. Inflammation of the whole brain.
Papilloedema. Swelling of the optic nerve seen with an ophthalmoscope.
Papillitis. Swelling of optic nerve due to 'inflammation'.
Para-. Alongside (e.g., paraventricular).
Paraplegia (paraparesis). Paralysis (weakness) of both legs.

Parkinsonism. The tremor and rigidity of Parkinson's disease.
Pes cavus. Very high arches to the feet.
Petit mal. A form of epilepsy; frequent episodes of detachment from surroundings.
Photophobia. Dislike of light.
Pia mater. The innermost layer of meninges.
Pineal gland. A structure lying in the centre of the skull, frequently calcified and visible on X-ray.
Plantar reflex. Toe movement on scratching the sole.
Plaques. Patches; usually applied to areas of demyelination in disseminated sclerosis.
Pneumoencephalography. See Air-encephalography.
Polioencephalitis. Brain stem infection by poliomyelitis virus.
Poly-. Many (e.g. polyneuritis, inflammation of many nerves).
Position (postural) sense. Knowledge of where each part of the body is without looking at it.
Posterior columns. Spinal cord tracts carrying position, vibration, and discriminative sensations.
Posterior horns. Part of spinal grey matter receiving sensory roots.
Pre-senile dementia. Cerebral atrophy in middle age.
Pressure cone. The forcing of brain tissue through a foramen, as a result of high pressure above, e.g. tentorial or cerebellar pressure cones.
Proptosis. Prominence of the eye with drooping of the lid.
Pseudohypertrophy. Apparent, but not true, enlargement.
Psychomotor epilepsy. Disturbance of behaviour due to epileptic discharges.
Psychoneurotic. Of psychological, not disease, origin.
Ptosis. Drooping of the eyelid.
Pyogenic. Causing the formation of pus.
Pyramidal cells, tracts. The pathways controlling voluntary movement; the upper motor neurones.

Quadriplegia. Paralysis of all four limbs (should be 'tetraplegia').
Queckenstedt test. Rise in lumbar C.S.F. pressure on compressing the jugular vein.

Reflex. An automatic response to a stimulus.
Relapse. A further attack of a disease.
Remission. A period of recovery from a disease.
Retro-bulbar. Behind the eye.
Rhinorrhoea. Running from the nose.
Rigidity. Stiffness due to equal resistance in all muscles.
Roots. Nerve fibres as they enter or leave the stem or cord.

Scanning (brain). Detecting the distribution of a radioactive substance in the brain.
Sclerosis. Hardening.
Scotoma. A patch of blindness.
Sella turcica. A saddle-shaped cavity at the base of the skull containing the pituitary gland.
Sensory. Concerned with feeling.
Sensory level. The point where sensation changes from abnormal to normal.
Shunt. A method of by-passing an obstruction to C.S.F. flow.
Space-occupying lesion. A tumour, or other growing lesion.
Spastic ataxia. A combination of spasticity and unsteadiness.
Spasticity. Increased tone (affecting some muscles more than others).
Spondylosis. Degenerative changes in bones and discs in the spine.
Status epilepticus. Fits following each other in rapid succession.
Stenosis. Narrowing.
Stereotaxis. Accurately placing small lesions in the depths of the brain.
Strabismus. A squint.
Stretch reflex. Contraction of muscle following its sudden stretching.
Stupor. Unconscious, but rousable.
Subarachnoid. Between arachnoid and pia.
Subdural. Between dura and arachnoid.
Sulci. Furrows on the surface of the brain.
Superficial reflex. Various muscle contractions following stimuli to the skin surface.
Symptomatic. Representing a disease process.
Syndrome. A collection of signs and symptoms recurring frequently enough to be recognisable.
Syrinx. A cavity in brain stem or cord.

Teichopsia. Flashes of light in migraine.
Tentorial herniation. Forcing part of the brain through the tentorial hiatus.
Tentorium. Tent-like sheet of dura separating cerebellum from cerebral hemispheres.
Tetraplegia. Paralysis of all four limbs.
Thecal space. Colloquial term applied to the space formed by the meninges containing C.S.F.
Tic. A recurrent spasm (e.g. tic douloureux).
Tinnitus. Ringing in the ears.
Todd's paralysis. Temporary paralysis of a part following a fit.
Tomography. Taking X-rays focused at different levels.
Tone. The tension present in muscle at rest.

Tonsils. In neurology refers to a part of the cerebellum.
Torticollis. Twisting of the neck to one side.
Tracts. Collection of nerve fibres having similar functions.
Trophic. Changes occurring in tissues which have lost their nerve supply.

Upper motor neurone. The motor cells and fibres running from the cerebral cortex to cranial nerve nuclei and anterior horn cells.

Vagus. Xth cranial nerve. Used to be called **pneumogastric.**
Ventricles. Cavities in the brain containing C.S.F.
Ventriculography. X-raying the ventricles by injecting air directly into them.
Vertigo. A sense of rotation.
Vestibular. Concerned with the labyrinth and its connections.
Vibration sense. Ability to detect tuning fork vibration.
Viral. Due to infection by a virus.

White matter. The parts of brain and spinal cord containing myelinated fibres.

Xanthochromic. Yellow coloured.

3 *THE STRUCTURE AND FUNCTION OF THE NERVOUS SYSTEM*

The nervous system is made up of the Central Nervous System, the Peripheral Nervous System and the Autonomic Nervous System. All three are intimately connected and the autonomic system has special functions which are dealt with separately at the end of the chapter.

The **Central Nervous System** (see Fig. 3.1) consists of (a) the **brain,** which includes the two **cerebral hemispheres,** the **brain stem,** and the **cerebellum,** and (b) the **spinal cord.** The brain occupies the interior of the skull and is continuous with the spinal cord at the **foramen magnum,** the largest opening in the base of the skull. The spinal cord then passes down the **vertebral canal,** which is a tube bounded in front by the vertebral bodies and behind by an arch formed by the laminae and spinous processes (Fig. 3.2).

The **Peripheral Nervous System** consists of (a) the **cranial nerves,** which arise from, or travel to, the brain stem, and (b) the **spinal nerves,** which travel to or from the spinal cord. Some peripheral nerves are purely **motor,** concerned only with the movement of muscles; others are purely **sensory,** carrying various sensations inwards to the central nervous system. Most, however, are mixed nerves, carrying fibres of each type. By repeatedly branching, the peripheral nerves carry their fibres to all parts and every organ of the body.

The Structure of Nervous Tissue

Nervous tissue consists of three main elements, **nerve cells, nerve fibres** and the supporting tissue, consisting of cells and fibres known as the **glia.** Each nerve cell has several processes, one of which is much larger than the others and becomes the nerve fibre. The cell and its fibre together constitute the **neurone** (Fig. 3.3). Fibres which serve a particular purpose tend to run together within the central nervous system in **tracts.** It is bundles of such fibres running from the cells in the brain stem or spinal cord to the muscles, skin or other organs that constitute the cranial and spinal peripheral nerves. Most fibres are clothed with a sheath of white substance called **myelin.** Where there are many cells together, or

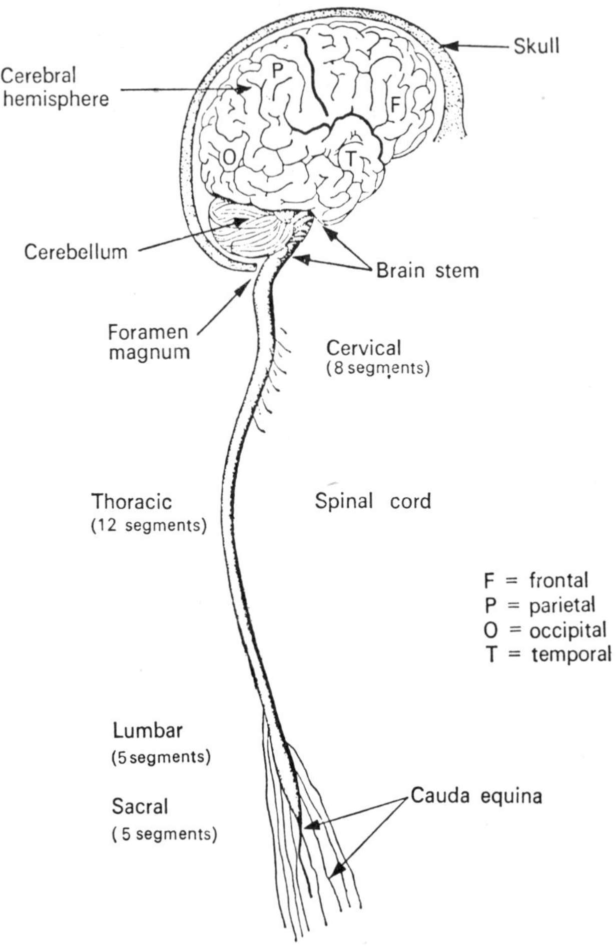

FIG. 3.1 The Central Nervous System. The spinal cord is considered to be divided into 8 cervical, 12 thoracic, 5 lumbar and 5 sacral segments, each of which sends off a pair of spinal nerves. These, together with the cranial nerves, constitute the peripheral nervous system.

when the fibres have no myelin sheath, the colour of the nervous tissue is dark and is referred to as **grey matter.** This forms the surface layer of the cerebral hemispheres (the cerebral **cortex**) and also the deeply placed **basal ganglia,** various nuclei in the brain stem, and the central portion of the spinal cord. Where there are many nerve fibres together the myelin sheaths cause the tissue to be

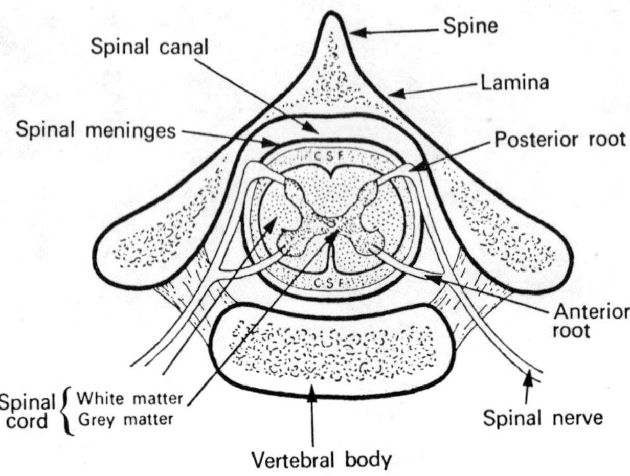

FIG. 3.2 The vertebral column cut across to show the spinal cord in the spinal canal, and the emerging nerve roots.

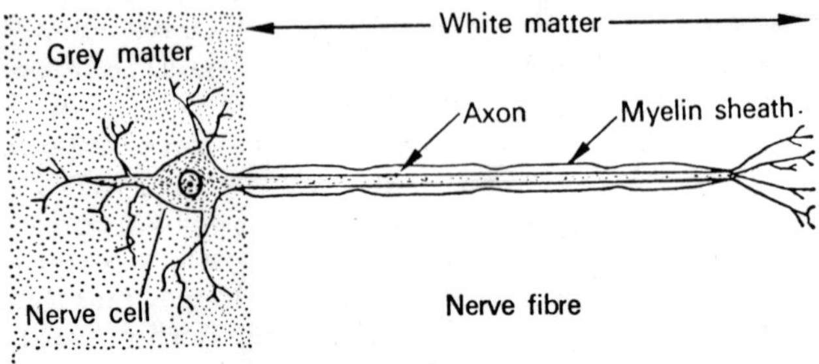

FIG. 3.3 Diagram illustrating the structure of a neurone.

pale and so to be called the **white matter.** It is the contrast of grey and white matter that gives the characteristic appearance to sections of brain and spinal cord.

The Coverings of the Central Nervous System

The skull is, of course, the main protection to the brain, but within the skull the brain is covered and further protected by three membranes, or **meninges.** The outer membrane, the **dura mater** (Fig. 3.4), is tough, has two layers and lines the skull, and by extending downwards through the foramen magnum also lines the vertebral canal. Between its layers inside the skull lie great venous sinuses. The dura is separated from the next membrane, a web-like

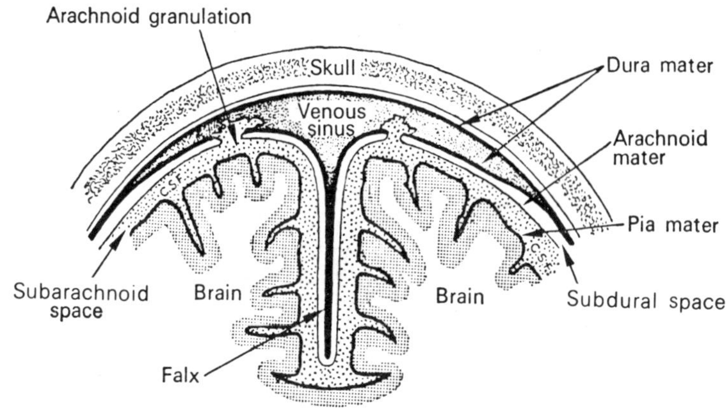

FIG. 3.4 Diagram to show the coverings of the brain. Note the two layers of dura mater, the venous sinuses lying in between.

tissue called the **arachnoid mater,** by a thin space crossed by fine blood vessels. The arachnoid loosely covers the brain and spinal cord, but is separated from the innermost of the three membranes, the **pia mater,** by a further space, the **subarachnoid space,** which contains the **cerebro-spinal fluid.** The pia is closely applied to all the many folds (**gyri**), and furrows (**sulci**), which characterise the surface of the brain. The cerebro-spinal fluid bathes the brain and spinal cord and acts as a cushion protecting them against the numerous jolts of every day life. The spinal cord is covered and protected by extensions of these same three meninges, and the dura and the arachnoid pass much lower down the vertebral canal than does the spinal cord itself, thus forming a sac in the lumbar region from which spinal fluid can be withdrawn (Chap. 20).

The Brain (Fig. 3.5)

The brain is divisible into several parts, the largest of which are the two cerebral hemispheres. These occupy the anterior and middle fossae of the skull. During development the surface of the brain becomes folded, forming the gyri, in between which are furrows, or sulci. These are not formed in a haphazard manner, but show the same pattern in each normal brain. The two hemispheres are separated in their upper parts by the median longitudinal fissure (Fig. 3.6). Anteriorly and posteriorly this separation is complete, but in the depths of the fissure centrally they are joined by a block of fibres called the **corpus callosum.** The dura forms a tough sheet which dips into the longitudinal fissure and is called the **falx** cerebri.

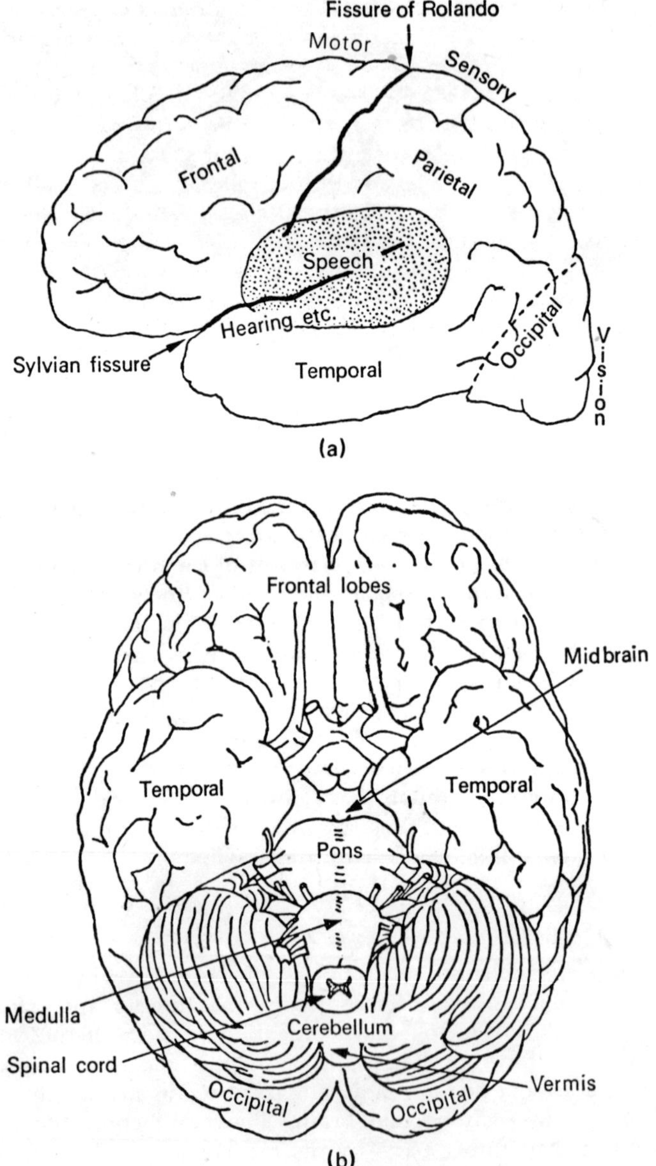

FIG. 3.5 (a) The outer, or lateral, surface of the left cerebral hemisphere showing its division into lobes and the areas having special functions. (b) The under, or basal, surface of the brain showing brain stem and cerebellum. The stem is cut across as it becomes continuous with the spinal cord.

Each hemisphere is somewhat artificially divided into **lobes.** The most anterior is the **frontal lobe** (Fig. 3.5). Damage to parts of this may produce personality change, and in its posterior part lie the cells controlling motor activity (i.e. movement) throughout the body. The frontal lobe ends at a well-marked sulcus named the **Fissure of Rolando,** posterior to which lies the **parietal lobe,** which is of major importance for the appreciation of sensation. Most posterior of all is the **occipital lobe.** Here the stimuli of vision are received. In front of the occipital lobe, but below the parietal lobe, lies the **temporal lobe,** separated to some extent from the posterior part of the frontal lobe by another deep fissure, the **Sylvian Fissure.** Stimuli of taste, sound, and smell are received by the temporal lobe and it has also the power of converting crude visual impressions into recognisable pictures and scenes.

The areas where the frontal, parietal and temporal lobes are joined is responsible for that special function which makes the human being different from the lower animals—the function of **speech.** This is controlled by the left hemisphere in all right-handed people and by the right hemisphere in many, but by no means all, left-handed people.

Deeply placed in the centre of the hemispheres to either side of the midline are the **basal ganglia** (or basal nuclei) (Fig. 3.6), of which the most important is the **thalamus.** These are vital sorting stations where messages passing to and from the hemispheres are collected and redistributed.

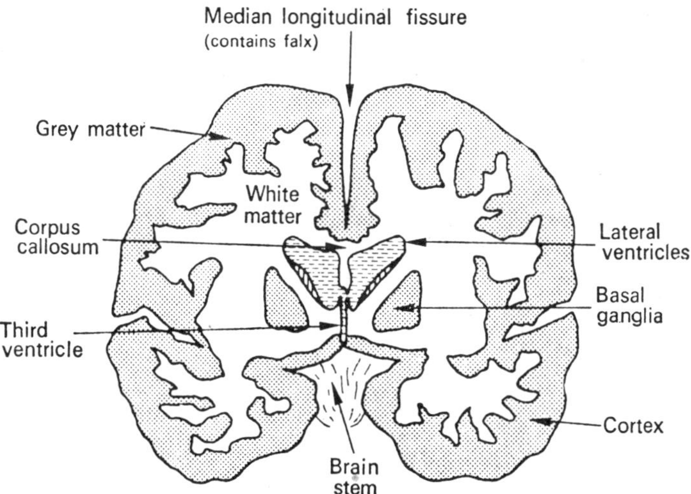

FIG. 3.6 Diagram of a cross section of the cerebral hemispheres to show the principal anatomical features.

Below the hemispheres and connected to them by two thick bunches of fibres, the cerebral peduncles, lies the **brain stem.** This is a single midline structure carrying all the nerve fibres passing between cerebral hemispheres, cerebellum, and spinal cord. It extends from the cerebral hemispheres to the foramen magnum, where it is continuous with the spinal cord. All cranial nerves, except the first, enter or arise from the brain stem. Its most superior portion is called the **midbrain,** and contains the nerve cells controlling eye movement. Below this lies the **pons,** and below that the **medulla oblongata,** which controls many vital functions such as swallowing, breathing and the action of the heart.

Above and behind the brain stem, but also joined to it, lies the **cerebellum.** This is separated from the cerebral hemispheres by a tough, tent-shaped sheet of meninges called the **tentorium.** This sheet divides the cavity of the skull into the anterior and middle

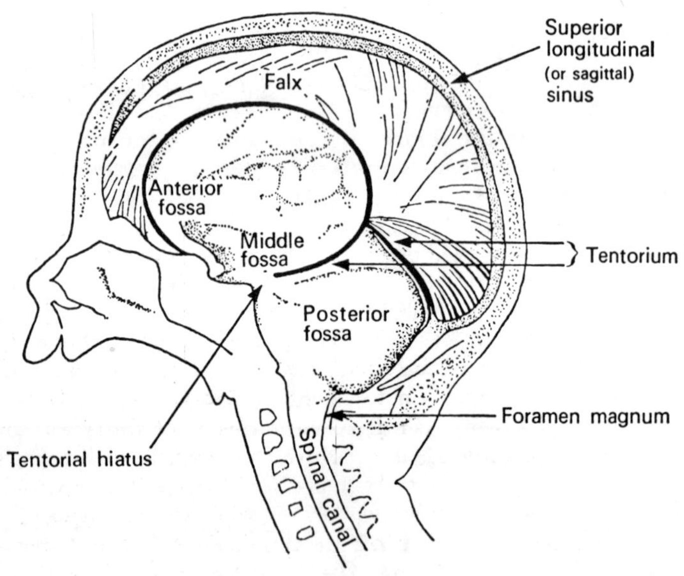

FIG. 3.7 Diagram to show the division of the skull into compartments by sheets of dura mater.

fossae above, and the posterior fossa below (Fig. 3.7). It has to have in it a large gap—the **tentorial hiatus,** through which the brain stem can pass. The cerebellum has two lateral lobes joined by a midline portion named the **vermis.** It is important in the co-ordination of all muscle movements, including walking, talking and in the control of muscle tone and of balance.

The Spinal Cord

The spinal cord runs down in the spinal canal from the foramen magnum to the level of the first lumbar vertebra. If it is cut across (Fig. 3.8), it can be seen that in the centre there is an H-shaped zone of grey matter surrounded by white matter. The more pointed limbs of the H are called the **posterior horns,** and the plumper limbs are the **anterior horns.** Though anatomically a continuous structure, it is convenient to divide the cord into **8** cervical, **12** thoracic, **5** lumbar and **5** sacral **segments.** Each segment receives sensory nerve roots and gives off motor nerve roots on either side. These **roots** join to become peripheral nerves, which pass out between the vertebrae, there being one more cervical pair than there are cervical vertebrae.

It has already been said that the cord is much shorter than the spine and the spinal canal, so that the lower spinal nerves have to become more and more vertical in their course to reach their points of exit (the root foraminae). Below L.1 there are so many passing in a downward direction to their exit foraminae in the lumbo-sacral region that they resemble a horse's tail and are called the **cauda equina** (Fig. 3.9)

The Ventricles and Spinal Fluid Pathways

The brain is not an entirely solid structure. Deep in each cerebral hemisphere is a cavity called the **lateral ventricle** (Fig. 3.6); these two ventricles are connected by foramina to a narrow centrally placed cavity, the **third ventricle.** From the posterior part of this a thin channel (the **aqueduct of Sylvius**) runs through the midbrain and widens below the cerebellum to form the **fourth ventricle** (Fig. 3.10). A very small channel continues from this down the spinal cord as its central canal while small apertures (**foramina**) in the fourth ventricle communicate with the subarachnoid space. The ventricles contain tufts of vascular tissue called the **choroid plexuses.** It is from these that the **cerebro-spinal fluid** is formed. This fluid passes from the lateral ventricles into the third ventricle, through the aqueduct to the fourth ventricle, and then out through the foramina in this ventricle to gain the subarachnoid space. It then flows upwards over the surface of the brain and into its fissures, and downwards through the foramen magnum over the surface of the spinal cord. At the base of the brain the meninges are so arranged that several pools, or cisterns, of fluid can collect, the most important of which is the **cisterna magna,** lying just behind the medulla and above the foramen magnum (Fig. 3.10). The spinal fluid is constantly circulating, and is re-absorbed into the bloodstream by **tufts of**

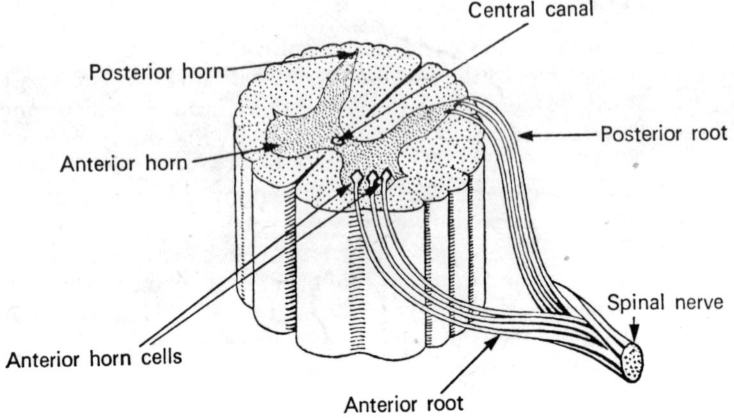

FIG. 3.8 A block section of the spinal cord.

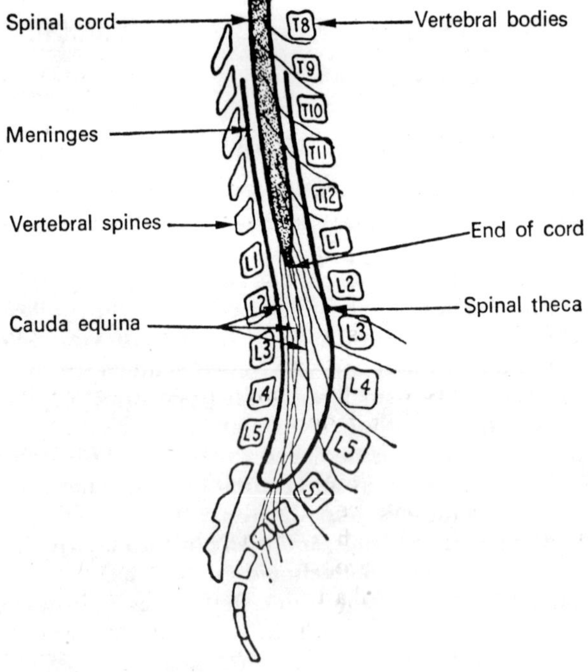

FIG. 3.9 Diagram of lateral view of lower end of spine. Note the meninges extend well below the end of the cord, forming a sac containing C.S.F. and the nerve roots of the cauda equina.

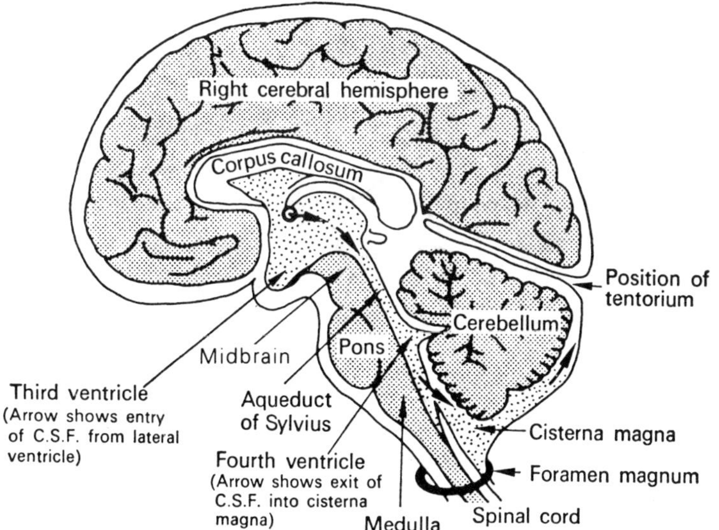

FIG. 3.10 Diagram of a section through the brain passing between the two cerebral and cerebellar hemispheres, and bisecting the brain stem and the C.S.F. pathways. The lateral ventricle cannot be seen as it is contained within the hemisphere.

arachnoid which lie on the superior surface of the cerebral hemispheres and project into the venous sinuses between the layers of the dura (Fig. 3.4).

The Blood Supply

The nervous system is almost more dependent on its blood supply than any other organ. If the brain cells are deprived of the oxygen in the blood for more than 3–4 minutes they will die, unless the needs of the cells have been reduced by lowering their temperature (hypothermia), when they may survive longer. The blood is carried to the brain by the two **internal carotid arteries** anteriorly, and by the two **vertebral arteries** posteriorly (read this in conjunction with Figs. 3.11 and 3.12). Each internal carotid artery divides inside the skull into the **anterior cerebral artery** and the **middle cerebral artery.** The anterior cerebral artery supplies most of the frontal lobe of the brain, and the middle cerebral artery supplies the rest of the frontal region and the parietal and part of the temporal lobes. The two vertebral arteries run up through channels in the cervical spine (in quite close contact with both vertebrae and discs), enter the skull at the foramen magnum, and then join together to form the **basilar artery.** This lies on the under surface of the brain stem, supplies

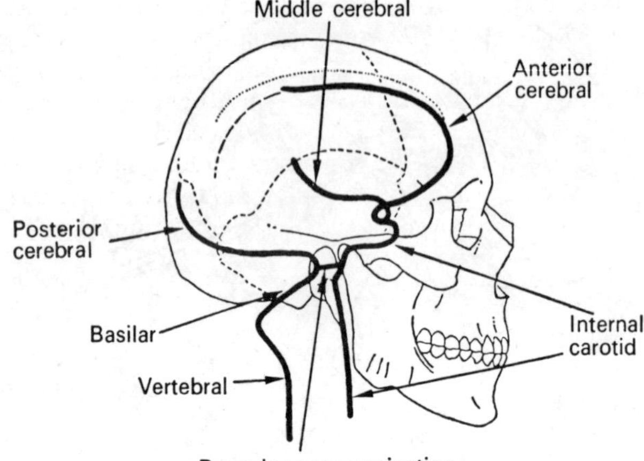

FIG. 3.11 The arteries supplying the brain. Lateral view of head and neck showing internal carotid and vertebral arteries and main branches.

through its branches both this vital structure and the cerebellum, and finally divides again into the two **posterior cerebral arteries,** which supply the occipital region of the cerebral hemispheres. The anterior and posterior parts of the cerebral circulation are not, however, completely separate. Each carotid artery is joined to the corresponding posterior cerebral artery by the **posterior communicating artery,** and the two anterior cerebral arteries are joined by a minute vessel, the **anterior communicating artery.** In this way,

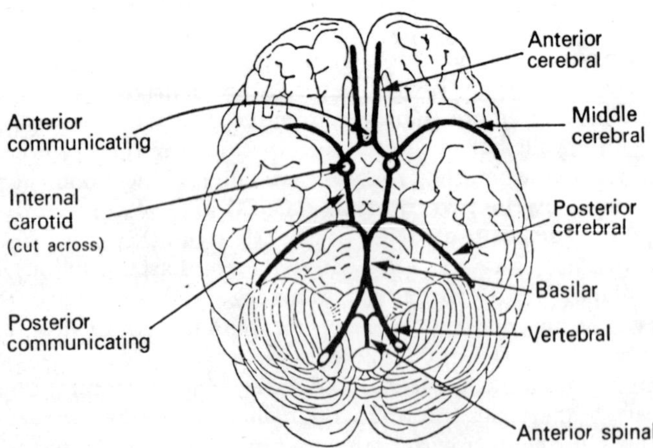

FIG. 3.12 Basal view of brain showing the Circle of Willis. Carotid and vertebral arteries have been cut across.

there is a continuous circle of vessels at the base of the brain—the **Circle of Willis**—and if for some reason the flow of blood through, for example, one carotid artery, stops, the appropriate area of the brain can still receive its supply from the other carotid, or even from the vertebrals, by means of this continuous circle.

The vertebral arteries give off vessels which run downwards and supply the spinal cord. Though reinforced by vessels entering with a few of the spinal nerve roots, the blood supply of the cord is a little precarious.

The Motor System (Fig. 3.13)

In the cerebral cortex in front of the Fissure of Rolando, there are thousands of motor nerve cells. These include large cells, shaped like pyramids, called **Betz cells** or **Pyramidal cells.** The cells which control movement of the legs are situated near the uppermost point of the hemisphere, and those which control the facial movements are in the inferior portion. The body is, therefore, represented upside down. The fibres originating from these cells in each hemisphere converge in the depths of the brain, and pass in a compact group between the basal nuclei to the cerebral peduncles and so on to the brain stem. There they **cross over to the other side,** and it is for this reason that a lesion of one hemisphere causes paralysis of the opposite side of the body. These fibres are called the **pyramidal fibres;** they run together as the pyramidal tracts, and together with their cells they constitute the **upper motor neurones.** Some pyramidal fibres end at the nuclei of the motor cranial nerves in the brain stem but the others pass down the lateral aspect of the spinal cord to end in relation to further motor cells which lie in the anterior horns of the grey matter in the spinal cord. From all these motor cells new neurones arise which carry impulses away from the central nervous system through the peripheral nerves to the muscles supplied from that particular segment. These are the **lower motor neurones.** There are upper and lower motor neurones for each motor activity, and it will be appreciated that the upper motor neurones run *entirely* within the brain and spinal cord, but apart from their cells the major part of the lower motor neurones lie outside the central nervous system

Voluntary movement is not a simple matter resulting merely from a series of impulses from pyramidal cells reaching appropriate muscles. Fibres arising from many other cerebral sources (frontal lobes, basal ganglia, brain stem) which are separate from the pyramidal cell system, and are called **extrapyramidal** fibres, together with further fibres from the **cerebellum,** all form tracts which bring influence to bear upon the cells of the lower motor

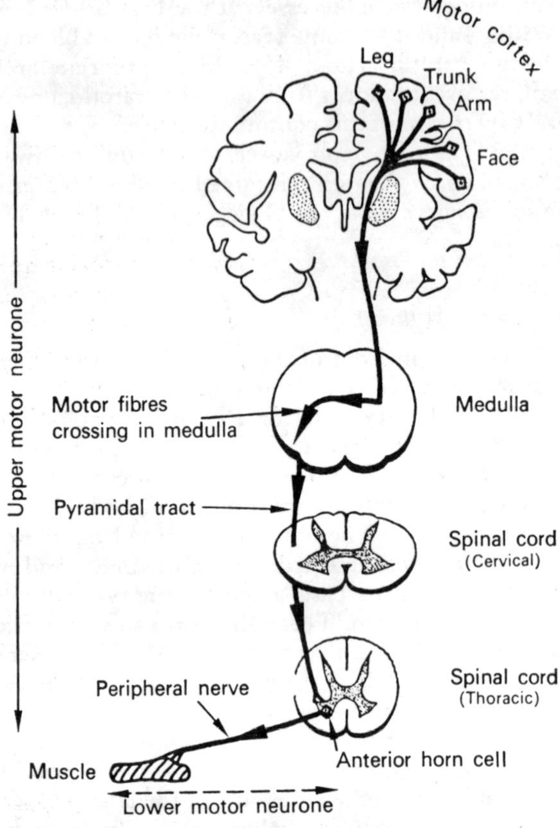

FIG. 3.13 Diagram of the motor pathways.

neurone, ensuring that when a muscle contracts it does so smoothly, adequately, not too little, not too much, and that the correct opposing muscles relax. Without such influences normal smooth movements would be impossible, and even the maintenance of posture and balance would be severely affected.

The Sensory System

Many forms of sensation are possible, but there are certain forms which are easy to examine and whose pathways through the nervous system have been well worked out. These include sensations of **pain, light touch, temperature, position, vibration,** and recognition of **shape, size,** and **texture.** In addition, the special senses of vision, hearing, smell, and taste have their own separate pathways.

In the skin, the muscles, and around the joints there are special types of nerve endings which respond to different types of stimulus, e.g. pain or heat. For these stimuli to be appreciated as one of the familiar sensations they must first travel back to the central nervous system. This they do either in the sensory cranial nerves (from the head), or in the spinal peripheral nerves (from the rest of the body).

As the sensory fibres near the spinal cord at each level they are separated from the motor fibres and form the **posterior nerve root,** which is entirely sensory (Fig. 3.14). They have their cells in a ganglion on this root, and these cells send another fibre to enter the postero-lateral part of the spinal cord. There is then a reorganisation of fibres which is of great importance in neurological diagnosis. The fibres carrying pain and temperature and some of those carrying light touch, pass their impulses on to second sensory neurones which then cross over to the opposite side of the cord. There they lie in its more anterior portion, and travel upwards through the cord and brain stem to the thalamus, in the **spinothalamic tract.** A further sensory neurone then carries the impulses to the **sensory cortex** in the cerebral hemisphere, which, it will be remembered, lies in the parietal lobe behind the Fissure of Rolando. Here again the body is represented upside down, the feet near the longitudinal fissure in the most superior part of the hemisphere.

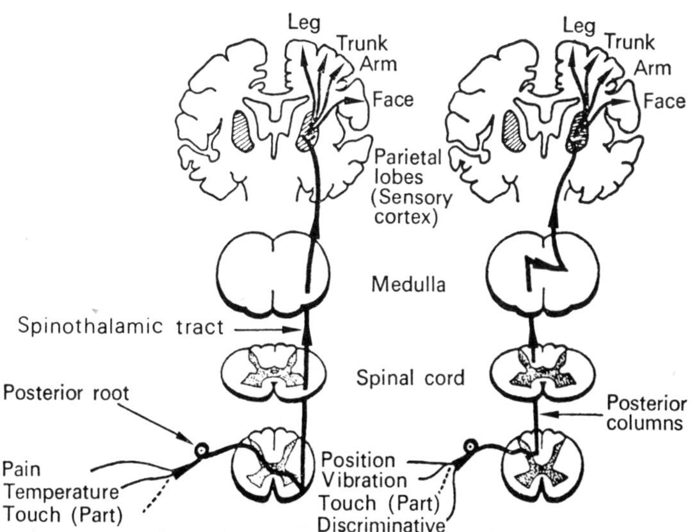

FIG. 3.14 The pathways by which different forms of sensation reach the brain.

Those fibres carrying position and vibration sense, some elements of touch, and discriminative sense, however, after entering the cord, turn directly upwards without crossing, and travel in two columns lying in the posterior aspect of the cord—the **posterior columns.** They have to cross at some stage and they do this in the brain stem, and then they too pass to the thalamus, so that at this site fibres for all sensations are together, and their messages can be passed on to the parietal cortex. It is thought that one becomes conscious of pain, temperature and vibration sensations when they reach the thalamic level, while other sensations are appreciated at the cortex, but these facts, and the exact method by which the different types of sensation travel, are still under discussion, and the process is infinitely more complex than suggested here. For many years, however, the ideas expressed above have been of practical value in locating a patient's lesion.

The anatomy of the cranial nerves differs in so many respects that it will be easier to deal with it briefly when considering lesions of these nerves.

Nerve Impulses and How They Travel

The nervous system works by electricity. A nerve cell gives off an electrical discharge which travels along the fibre, exciting another discharge either in the cell of a connecting neurone, or in the muscle or organ to which it runs. The discharge in (e.g.) the muscle causes it to contract. Similar electrical discharges carry sensations inwards to the brain or spinal cord, and in the brain there is constant electrical activity as messages are passed from one part to another, and either 'filed away' as memory, or 'passed for action' by producing some movement, or sight, or smell. These electrical waves are, of course, minute, but modern machines can detect them and amplify them so that they can be recorded.

The Reflexes

In simplest terms, a **reflex** is a reaction that occurs automatically. Examples are the involuntary blink during a flash-light photograph, or the smart withdrawal of a foot from a piece of holly under the bedclothes. For any reflex to occur, there must first be a **stimulus,** then a **sensory** nerve to carry the stimulus, a connection between a sensory nerve and a motor nerve, a **motor** nerve running to the part of the body which responds, and a muscle or some other structure to respond. This circuit is termed the **reflex arc** (Fig. 3.15), and if any point in it is damaged that reflex, when tested, will be absent. Many of these arcs also come under influences from the

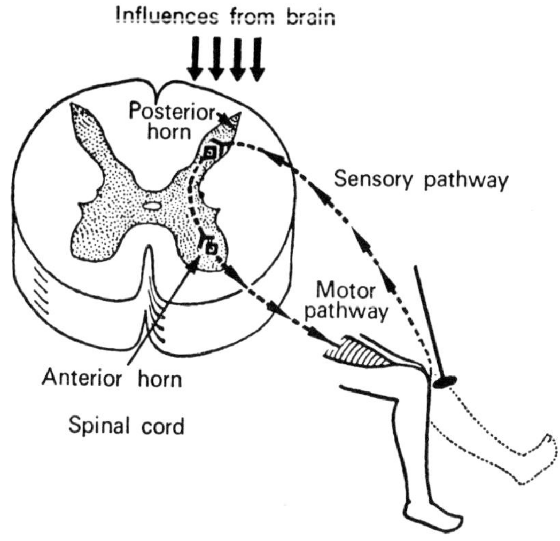

FIG. 3.15 Diagram of a reflex arc. The reflex illustrated is the knee jerk.

brain which alter the response in some way. If the pathways from the brain to the arc are damaged, so that their influences are absent, there may be a great difference in the response obtained. A number of important reflexes are used in neurological examination.

Pupillary Reflexes. When light is shone into the eye, or the patient looks at a near object, the pupil normally becomes smaller.

Stretch Reflexes (Tendon Reflexes). Suddenly stretching a muscle (e.g. by striking its tendon) causes that muscle to contract and part of the limb to move.

Superficial Reflexes. Stroking the abdominal skin causes the abdominal muscles to contract—the **abdominal reflexes.** Scratching the sole of the foot normally causes the big toe to flex (Fig. 3.16)—a **flexor plantar reflex.** In disease the toe may go up instead—an **extensor plantar,** or **Babinski, reflex.**

Conditioned Reflexes. These have developed as a result of training and previous experience, e.g. salivation at the sight or smell of an appetising dish; the movement to put on the foot-brake by car-drivers when travelling as passengers; or the straightening of caps, etc., at the approach of the Senior Nursing Officer.

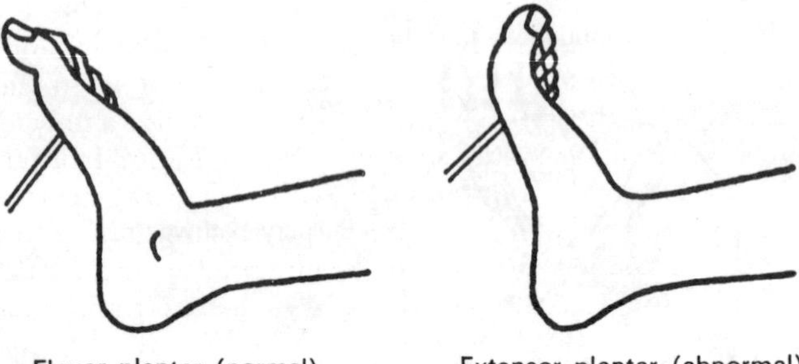

FIG. 3.16 The plantar reflex.

THE AUTONOMIC NERVOUS SYSTEM

We control, by will, the movements of our limbs, but the movements of the intestines, the secretion of glands, and the changes in the blood pressure, take place automatically, and are under the control of the autonomic nervous system. This system can be divided into two distinct parts—the **sympathetic system** and the **parasympathetic system.**

The Sympathetic System

Fibres arising in the brain stem pass down the cervical cord to small lateral projections in the grey matter of the 8th cervical to the 2nd lumbar segments. From these 'lateral horns' fibres leave the cord with the anterior roots at each level, but soon split and enter one of a series of **sympathetic ganglia** which lie in a vertical chain on the posterior wall of the thoracic and abdominal cavities on either side of the spinal column. More fibres leave these ganglia and rejoin the peripheral nerve and travel to all organs and vessels of the body. Those going to the head pass into the largest and most highly placed ganglion, the superior cervical or **stellate ganglion,** and then travel in the sheath of the carotid artery to enter the skull.

Activity of the sympathetic nervous system dilates the pupils, constricts the blood vessels of the skin and so cools it, decreases peristalsis, increases sweating and raises the blood sugar. You will recognise that many of these features are the symptoms of fear, and indeed they can be reproduced by injecting **adrenaline.** This substance is secreted in the body by the **adrenal medulla,** and the adrenal gland is closely connected with sympathetic activity, and with emotional responses. Paralysis of the sympathetic produces the opposite effects.

The Parasympathetic System

Some of the parasympathetic cells lie in the brain stem, and others in the sacral region of the spinal cord. The fibres from the brain stem travel with the IIIrd, VIIth, IXth, and Xth cranial nerves to the pupils, salivary glands, thoracic and abdominal organs, and those from the sacral region travel with the sacral nerves to the pelvic organs, especially the bladder and rectum. The Xth cranial nerve, the **vagus,** is the largest autonomic nerve and its parasympathetic fibres are distributed throughout the chest and abdominal organs.

Parasympathetic activity constricts the pupil, dilates skin vessels, increases salivation and peristalsis, and makes the bladder contract. It is stimulated by **acetyl-choline** and paralysed by **atropine.**

The two systems work together and the function of almost every organ requires some degree of action of each. The autonomic system is immensely complex and much less is certain about it than is the case for the rest of the nervous system.

This chapter describes the normal. Now we must consider how the nervous system behaves when it is damaged or diseased, and the next chapter deals with lesions as seen when examining patients.

4 *CLINICAL SIGNS OF DAMAGE TO NERVOUS TISSUE*

When a disease strikes an organ, some cells are totally **destroyed**; some are partially **damaged,** later to recover; some are **'irritated'** into abnormal activity; and some are left untouched. In the nervous system destruction results in total **paralysis** and/or total **loss of sensation**; damage causes paralysis, etc. at first, but considerable recovery later; irritation produces a variety of symptoms: if motor cells in the brain are involved, there are **convulsions**; if sensory nerves, there is **pain** or **tingling.** Whatever causes the damage, the nervous system can produce only a limited number of abnormal symptoms and signs, but exactly how these are distributed throughout the body depends entirely upon where the damaged area lies.

This chapter first describes in general terms the results of lesions of the motor and sensory systems, and then deals with those special features arising from damage to particular areas which make it possible to locate lesions fairly accurately.

Lesions of the Motor System

Damage to motor cells and fibres produces muscle **weakness,** muscle **wasting** and alterations in muscle **tone** (i.e. the degree of tension felt in a muscle at rest). The state of tone influences the behaviour of the tendon reflexes. The abnormalities found differ according to whether the lesion affects the upper motor neurone and lies between the cerebral cortex and the anterior horn cell, or the lower motor neurone and lies between the anterior horn cell and the muscle itself. The differences are as follows (Fig. 4.1):

Upper Motor Neurone Lesions	Lower Motor Neurone Lesions
Wasting slight	**Wasting** very marked
Weakness of any degree	**Weakness** usually marked
Tone increased (i.e. spastic)	**Tone** decreased (i.e. flaccid)
Tendon reflexes exaggerated	**Tendon reflexes** absent
Plantar reflexes extensor	**Plantar reflexes** flexor
Flexor spasms common	**Flexor spasms** do not occur
Fasciculation absent	**Fasciculation** common if cells involved

In addition to this, however, lesions of the other systems, extrapyramidal and cerebellar, which influence motor activity, cause abnormalities of their own (Fig. 4.2):

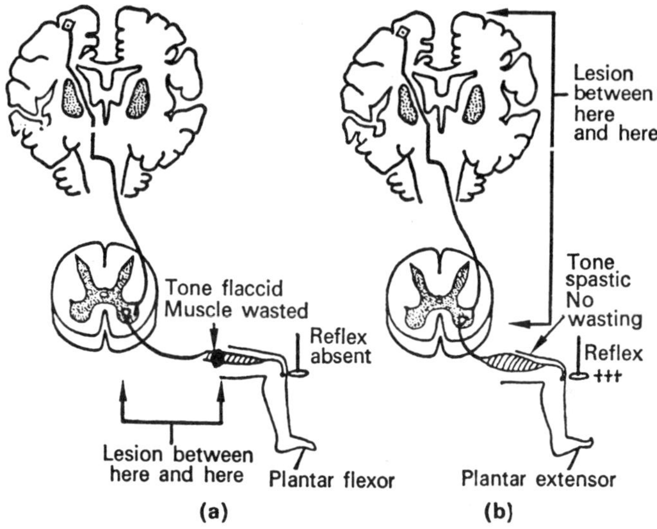

FIG. 4.1 Lesions of the motor system and the effects upon muscle tone and reflexes. (a) Lower and (b) upper motor neurone lesions.

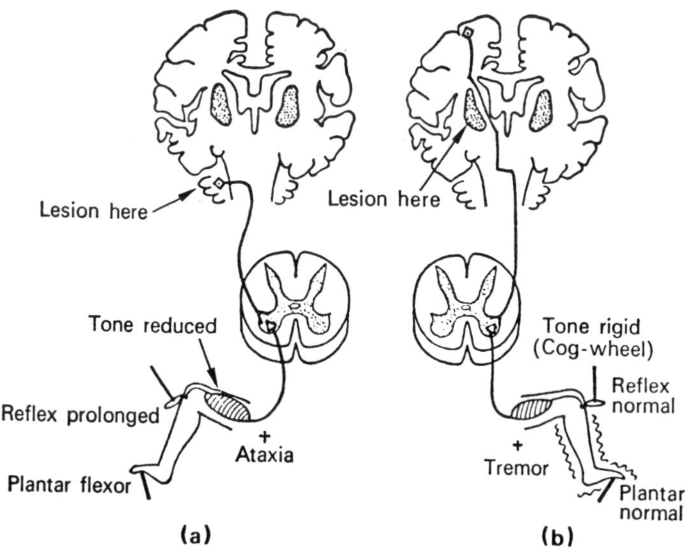

FIG. 4.2 Lesions of the motor system and the effects upon muscle tone and reflexes. (a) Cerebellar and (b) extrapyramidal lesions.

Extrapyramidal Lesions	Cerebellar Hemisphere Lesions
Wasting and weakness slight	**Wasting and weakness** absent
Tone jerkily increased, i.e. cog-wheel rigidity	**Tone** decreased
Tendon reflexes suppressed by rigidity	**Tendon reflexes** reduced
Plantar reflexes flexor	**Plantar reflexes** flexor
Tremor present at rest, reduced by movement	**Tremor** absent at rest, produced by movement (intention tremor)
No **ataxia**	Marked **ataxia**

Lesions of the Sensory System

Damage to sensory fibres causes loss of that particular sensation over the area from which the particular fibres have come. Loss of pain sensation is called **analgesia** (impairment = hypoalgesia); loss of light touch, **anaesthesia** (impairment = hypoaesthesia). Unusual sensitiveness is called **hyperalgesia** and **hyperaesthesia** respectively. Inability to appreciate the size and shape of an object is called **astereognosis,** and other forms of sensory impairment are described in full, e.g. 'loss of position sense'. See Fig. 4.3 to illustrate sensory abnormalities.

Postural Ataxia and Cerebellar Ataxia

If a patient has lost the sense of position in a limb, he cannot tell where that limb is unless he can see it. This causes an unsteadiness which is very severe when the eyes are closed, or when it is dark, but relatively slight at other times. On trying to place the finger on the nose, or the heel on the knee of the opposite leg he misses his object completely when the eyes are shut. This contrasts with cerebellar ataxia where there is a wavering unsteadiness which is much the same whether the eyes are open or shut, but accuracy of placing is not affected.

LOCATING THE LESION

Disease does not often pick out one group of fibres alone. Many permutations and combinations of the abnormalities described are possible and it is by discovering which particular combination is present in a given patient that the doctor is able to determine the site of the lesion.

As the cranial nerves lie in a small area and have special functions, signs that one or other of them is damaged narrows down the possible site of the lesion very greatly. These signs will now be described followed by an outline of the distribution of motor and sensory abnormalities produced by lesions in other parts of the system.

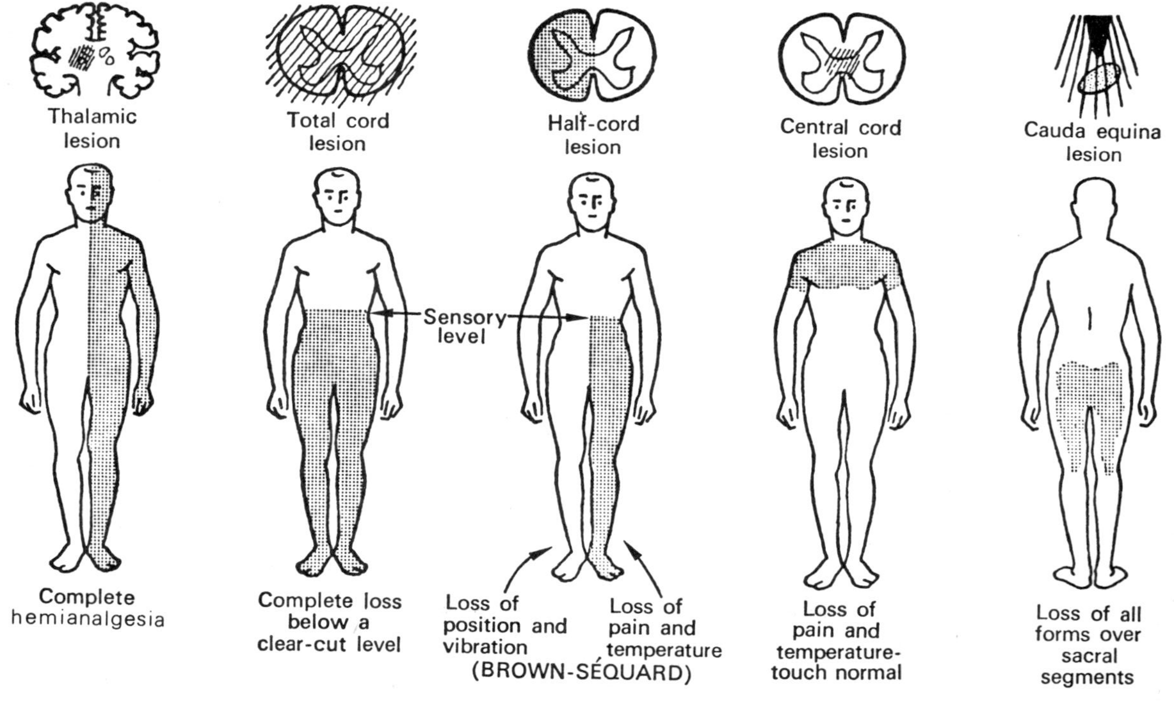

FIG. 4.3 Common patterns of sensory abnormality. The upper diagrams show the situation of the lesion; the lower, the distribution of the sensory loss.

Lesions of the Cranial Nerves (Fig. 4.4)

I The Olfactory Nerve. Fine filaments run from the nose, through a thin plate in the skull, to the olfactory bulb under the frontal lobe. These are often damaged after head injury, the result being loss of the sense of smell (**anosmia**) in one or both nostrils.

II The Optic Nerve. Rays of light pass through the lens of each eye and are focused on to special light-sensitive cells—the rods and cones—in the **retina.** The **cones,** sensitive to colour and bright light, lie mainly in one small area, the **macula.** The **rods** are more

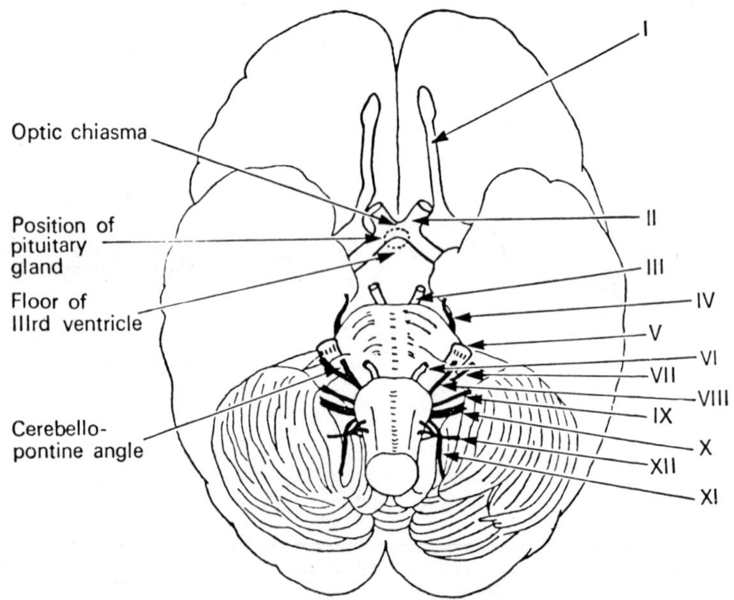

FIG. 4.4 The under or basal surface of the brain showing the origin of the cranial nerves.

widespread and are sensitive to weaker light. The rods and cones are connected to nerve fibres which run together and leave the eye as the **optic nerve.** With an ophthalmoscope their point of exit can be seen as a pale moon-like area called the **optic disc.** The amount of the outside world visible to each eye is termed the **field of vision,** its outer half being the temporal field, and its inner half the nasal field. Light from the temporal field falls on the nasal half of the retina, and from the nasal field on the temporal retina (Fig. 4.5). The nerve fibres arising from these two halves remains separate in the optic nerves. After the two nerves have left the orbits and entered the skull, they come together to form an X-like structure, the **optic chiasma,** which lies below the third ventricle and above the pituitary gland. Here the fibres from each nasal retina cross over to join the fibres from the temporal retina of the other eye. These two sets of fibres then form the **optic tracts,** which pass around the brain stem, and from which further fibres enter the cerebral hemispheres and spread out as the **optic radiations** to reach the **occipital cortex.** By this rearrangement of fibres at the chiasma, all impulses from the *right*-hand side of the field of vision (which stimulate the *left*-hand side of each retina) run in the *left* optic tract to the *left* cerebral hemisphere and the *left* occipital cortex (Fig. 4.5).

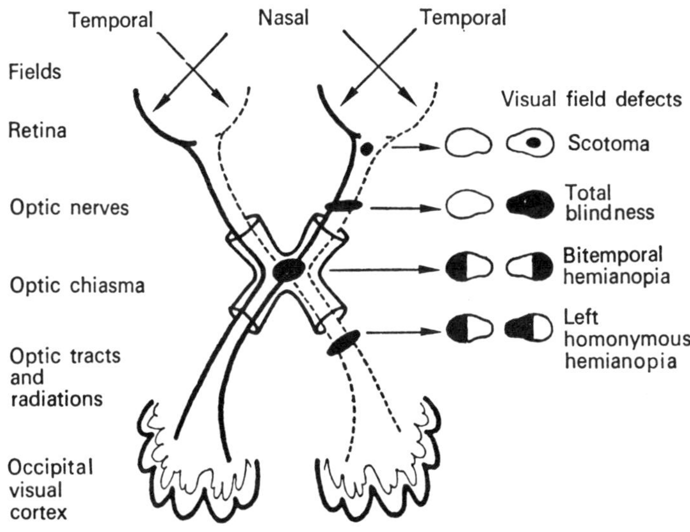

FIG. 4.5 The visual pathways, and common lesions. On the left are listed the anatomical divisions. The black marks show the site of various lesions, and the visual field defects which result are shown on the right.

Any lesion of the visual pathways results in some degree of blindness but how severe this is, and how much of the visual fields are affected, depends upon the exact site of the lesion. As a result of this arrangement of the fibres it is possible to locate the trouble fairly accurately (Fig. 4.5). A lesion of one optic nerve produces blindness of that eye alone, the other being unaffected. A small lesion inside an optic nerve produces a patch of blindness in the centre of the field of vision—the so-called **central scotoma.** Total destruction of the chiasma causes total blindness, but the common lesions at this site affect the central part of the chiasma. It is here that the fibres from the nasal halves of the retina cross each other, and this results in blindness in the temporal halves of the visual fields—**bitemporal hemianopia.** A lesion anywhere behind the chiasma, however, whether in optic tract, radiations, or occipital cortex, will affect the temporal field of one eye, and the nasal field of the other—an **homonymous hemianopia,** and always on the side opposite to the lesion.

By using an **ophthalmoscope,** it can be seen if the optic nerve is white and shrunken (**optic atrophy**), or if it is red and swollen. The latter is due to high pressure inside the skull, is called **papilloedema,** is common in brain tumours, and is one of the most important of all neurological signs.

III, IV, VI The Oculomotor, Trochlear and Abducent Nerves. These three nerves work together and control the muscles that move the eyes. The VIth nerve supplies the muscle which moves

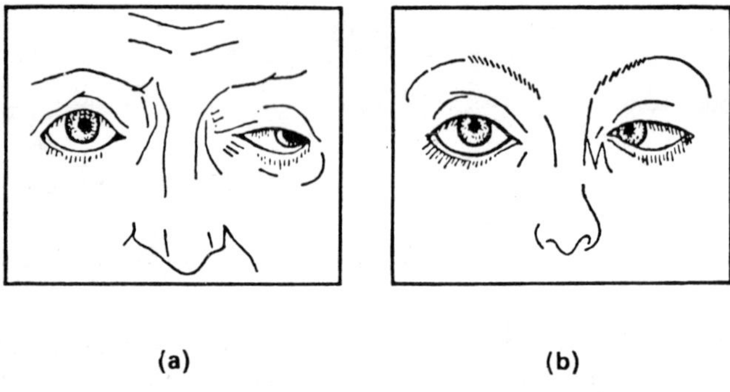

FIG. 4.6 (a) IIIrd nerve paralysis on left. Patient looking straight ahead, left eye wanders out, pupil dilates, lid droops; (b) VIth nerve paralysis on right. Patient trying to look to right, right eye cannot move outwards.

the eye outwards; the IIIrd and IVth nerves govern all other movements. The IIIrd also carries autonomic fibres which control the size of the pupil. Damage to the IIIrd nerve causes the lid to droop (**ptosis**); the pupil to dilate; and the eye to deviate outwards, (Fig. 4.6). VIth nerve damage, on the other hand, paralyses outward movement and the eye usually turns inwards (Fig. 4.6b). IVth nerve damage rarely occurs by itself. If, due to weakness of a muscle, eye movement gets 'out-of-step' light falls on different parts of the two retinae and causes double vision (**diplopia**). By looking for squints, testing eye movement and seeing in which position diplopia occurs, we can work out which nerve is damaged.

V The Trigeminal Nerve. Sensations from the face and front of the tongue run back in three divisions of the Vth nerve which join to enter its large ganglion (the **Gasserian ganglion**) in the base of the skull. The fibres then pass on as the trigeminal root to the brain stem. The nerve also has a small motor branch which supplies muscles used in chewing. Vth nerve damage (Fig. 4.7) causes sensory loss over one side of the face, one eye, the front of the tongue and scalp, but not over the angle of the jaw, or the occiput. The **corneal reflex** (blinking on both sides when one eye is touched) is absent.

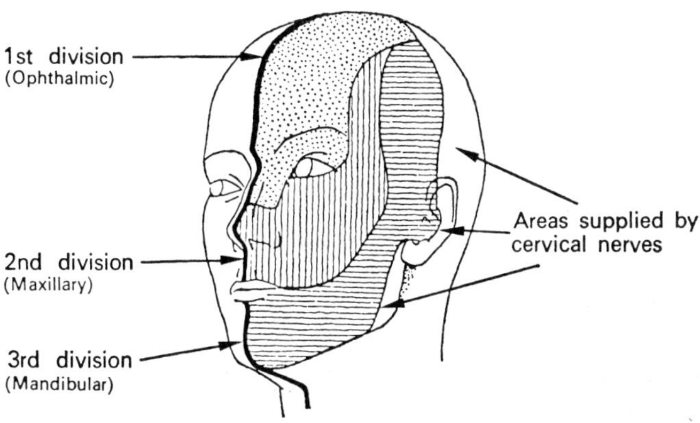

FIG. 4.7 Areas of the face supplied by the three divisions of the left trigeminal nerve.

VII The Facial Nerve. This is the motor nerve to all the **facial muscles.** Its upper motor neurones run from the opposite cerebral cortex to the pons, where its nucleus lies, very near to the VIth nerve nucleus. The nerve itself leaves the brain stem close to the Vth and VIIIth nerves in the angle between the cerebellum and pons, and travels to the face through a canal in the middle ear, taking with it autonomic fibres to control secretion of **tears** and **saliva.** It is joined by the sensory fibres of **taste.**

An upper motor lesion paralyses the opposite side of the mouth (Fig. 4.8a). A lower motor neurone lesion (i.e. the nerve itself) paralyses the whole of the face on the same side as the lesion (Fig. 4.8b).

VIII The Acoustic Nerve. This nerve, a special sensory nerve, is made up of two parts, one arising from the **cochlea** in the inner ear, and carrying impulses of sound, and the other arising from the **semicircular canals,** and carrying information regarding the rate and direction of head movement, which greatly influences **balance.**

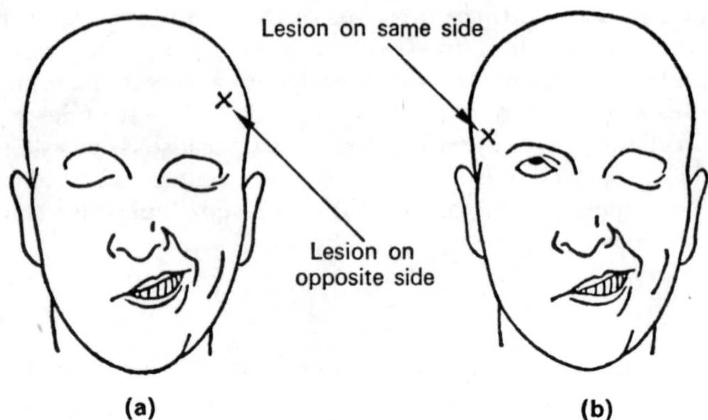

FIG. 4.8 Types of facial paralysis (a) right upper motor neurone weakness (lower face only); (b) right lower motor neurone weakness (upper and lower face affected).

Damage to the cochlear portion produces deafness. Partial lesions cause ringing noises (**tinnitus**). Lesions of the vestibular (labyrinthine) portion cause attacks of rotational giddiness (**vertigo**), vomiting and severe disturbance of balance. Lesions of both portions frequently occur together.

IX, X The Glossopharyngeal and Vagus Nerves. These two nerves arise from the medulla and between them control the movements of the **palate** and **pharynx**; in addition the IXth nerve carries sensation from the back of the tongue and throat, and the Xth nerve controls movement of the **vocal cords.** The vagus is also the largest autonomic nerve, and supplies these fibres to all the thoracic and abdominal organs. Damage to these nerves causes difficulty in swallowing, **nasal speech** due to palatal paralysis, and **hoarseness** if the vocal cords are paralysed. Damage to the vagus may alter heart rate and intestinal activity.

XI The Spinal Accessory Nerve. The roots of this nerve arise in the cervical region and travel upwards into the skull before leaving it again to supply the **trapezius** and **sternomastoid** muscles. Damage results in inability to shrug the shoulders and difficulty in turning the head to one side or bending it forwards.

XII The Hypoglossal Nerve. The last cranial nerve runs from the medulla to the muscles of the **tongue.** Damage to one nerve results in wasting of that half of the tongue (Fig. 4.9) and when it is protruded the normal side pushes it over towards the weak side. Bilateral

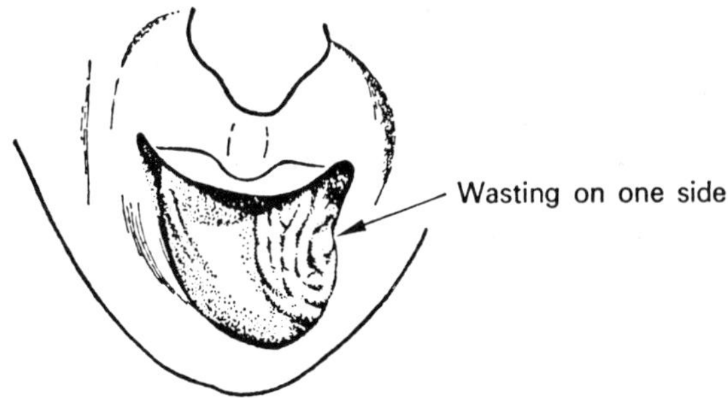

FIG. 4.9 Effect on tongue of paralysis of left hypoglossal (XIIth) nerve.

paralysis results in inability to move the tongue which, of course, causes gross disturbance of speech.

Lesions of the Cerebral Hemisphere

A lesion of one hemisphere shows its effects upon the opposite side of the body. The abnormalities produced depend upon (a) which lobe or lobes are involved, (b) how large the lesion is, and (c) how deep it extends. **Destruction** of the **motor area** in the posterior part of the frontal lobe produces a **hemiplegia**; a parietal lobe lesion (**sensory area**) produces loss of **position** and **discriminative** sensation on the opposite side; and a lesion in the **occipital** lobe produces a **homonymous hemianopia.** In the anterior parts of the frontal or temporal lobes, a small lesion may escape notice, though some produce disturbances of personality. A cerebral haemorrhage is a typical destructive lesion.

An **irritative** lesion which affects the cortex of the frontal, parietal or temporal lobes may produce **convulsions** involving part or the whole of the opposite half of the body. If these attacks start as twitching at one point which spreads throughout the body, they are then called **Jacksonian fits.** The same type of irritation in the visual cortex can produce vague flashes of light; in the temporal lobe, hallucinations of smell, or taste, or memory, and sometimes even quite clear visual pictures. A cerebral tumour is a typical irritative lesion at first, but, of course, as it grows larger it becomes destructive as well.

In the cerebral cortex the cells serving, for instance, the leg, are a long way away from those serving the face, but all fibres must come together as they reach the depths of the brain (see Fig. 3.13). In the internal capsule, therefore, a 5 mm lesion can cause a total hemiplegia, whereas on the surface of the brain one of 50 mm might merely cause weakness of one hand.

Lesions of the Cerebellum

Fibres from the cerebellum either stay on the same side, or if they cross the midline, they cross back again shortly afterwards. As a result a lesion of one side of the cerebellum will cause **ataxia** down the *same* side of the body, together with loss of tone, reduction of reflexes and a tendency to reel to that side when walking. Lesions of the cerebellar **vermis** cause **ataxia** when walking not found when the patient is lying down.

Lesions of the Spinal Cord (see Figs. 3.14 and 4.3)

Complete destruction of the cord at any point produces **paralysis** and **loss of sensation** of all those parts of the body which have their supply from nerves leaving or entering the cord **below the level** of the lesion. A lesion in the neck paralyses the arms, legs and respiratory muscles, but if it is in the thoracic cord, the arms will be entirely normal. The exact level of the lesion is usually worked out from the **sensory level,** i.e. the point where loss of sensation changes to normal sensation.

When there is partial cord damage, however, owing to the arrangement of sensory fibres, interesting signs are produced. Damage to one lateral half of the cord will affect (a) one pyramidal tract, producing paralysis on that side below the lesion; (b) one side of the posterior columns, causing loss of vibration and position sense on that side below the lesion; and (c) one spinothalamic tract. This causes loss of pain and temperature sense below the lesion, but as these fibres will have crossed from the other side of the cord, the sensory loss will be on the other side of the body. This combination of signs is called the **Brown-Séquard syndrome.** It puzzles patients greatly who cannot understand why, when one leg is weak, it is the other that feels numb.

If the lesion lies in the centre of the cord, it is possible for the pyramidal, posterior columns and spinothalamic tracts to escape, but it will involve the sensory fibres which *at that level* are crossing from their point of entry to join the opposite spinothalamic tract. Those crossing above or below are preserved. This produces an area of loss of pain and temperature on the skin on both sides, with normal sensation above and below. However, as many touch fibres travel up in the undamaged posterior columns, the remarkable situation may arise where a light touch may still be felt in an area where pain sense is absent. This is called **dissociated anaesthesia.**

Lesions of the Peripheral Nerves

Practically all peripheral nerves are mixed nerves. Each has a definite muscle or group of muscles to supply, and an area of skin from which to carry sensation. Damage to one nerve, therefore, results in weakness of a particular group of muscles and a patch of analgesia and anaesthesia. The neurologist has to learn the supply areas for each nerve to be able to recognise the one responsible. Sometimes however it is the ends of many nerves which are diseased at the same time. There is then both weakness and sensory loss in the periphery of all four limbs. This situation is found in polyneuritis, also called peripheral neuritis, or polyneuropathy (see p. 114).

Disturbances of Speech

A human being can speak or write, or understand what he hears or reads only if the so-called **'speech area'** of his brain is functioning correctly. This usually lies on the **left** side, even in left-handed people; but whereas all right-handed people have their speech centre on the left, a proportion (less than half) of those who are left-handed, have it on the right. It is situated in the lower and posterior part of the frontal lobe and the immediately adjacent parts of the parietal and temporal lobes. A lesion here causes what is known as **dysphasia,** or if it is complete, **aphasia.** The patient finds that he cannot form proper words or sentences, forgets the names of common objects, uses wrong words, or uses the same word over and over again, and has to make long-winded phrases to get over the failure to recall a name (e.g. a watch is called 'a thing to tell the time with'). The further forward in this area of the brain the lesion lies, the more difficulty there is in expressing his thoughts; the further back, the more difficulty in understanding what others say, or in reading, though hearing and sight may be normal.

For speech to be clear, however, the muscles of the tongue, the throat, the larynx and the face must work together properly. If there is disease of these muscles, or inco-ordination of their action, pronunciation becomes distorted and slurred, the words indistinct, and resembling drunken speech, yet the right words are used and the thoughts are correctly expressed. This is called **dysarthria,** and the lesion responsible may be anywhere from the cerebellum and the brain stem to the muscles producing speech themselves.

The distinction of these two types of speech defect is of great importance, for dysphasia must *always* means a lesion of the cerebral hemisphere, while dysarthria is usually due to a lesion 'below the tentorium'.

If the larynx and vocal cords are diseased the voice becomes hoarse or sinks to a whisper. This is dysphonia.

If *no attempt* is made to speak at all the term mutism is used.

5 *TRAUMA*

The skull and the vertebral column form such an excellent protection for the central nervous system that, though nervous tissue is very delicate, quite a severe injury is required for the brain or spinal cord to be damaged. Bone strength, thickness and resilience do, however, vary in different people and are influenced by age and the presence of disease. A small child may fall down a flight of stairs without turning a hair, while an old lady may merely need to bump her head on a mantelpiece to cause quite serious intracranial trouble.

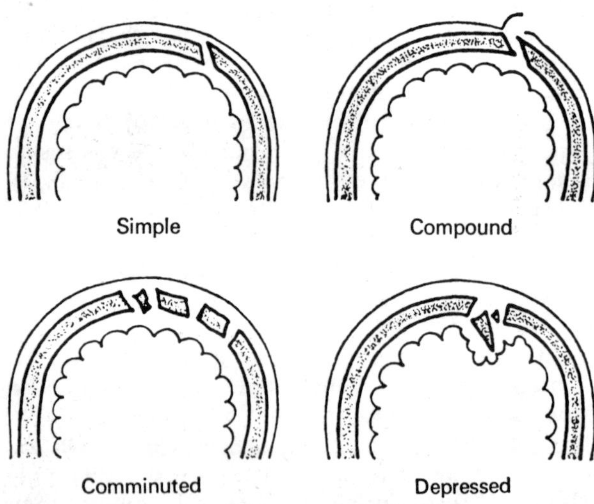

FIG. 5.1 The different types of skull fracture.

HEAD INJURIES

A **closed** head injury is one where, though the skull may be fractured, the coverings of the brain remain intact; in an **open** head injury the brain or meninges are exposed.

Fractures of the Skull (Fig. 5.1)

Skull fractures may occur either in the vault or across the base. They may be (a) simple **fissure** fractures, cracks with no break in the skin; (b) **compound** fractures, when the scalp is also breached; (c) more extensive **comminuted** fractures, the bone being broken into several pieces; or (d) **depressed** fractures, the most troublesome, when a piece of bone is driven inwards.

The fracture itself is of very little importance. The danger lies in damage to the underlying structures—the meninges, the blood vessels, and, of course, the brain—and because of this the position of the fracture is important. A frontal fracture may pass through the frontal sinuses and breach the dura. This allows a pathway to form between the nose and the interior of the skull so that CSF can escape down the nose (**CSF rhinorrhoea**). This might not be too serious, but it also allows air or infection to enter the skull. If this happens there is constant danger of recurrent attacks of meningitis. When the base of the skull is fractured, the petrous bones may be damaged. They contain the inner ear, and a fractured base may allow both blood and CSF to escape through the ears (**CSF otorrhoea**), and infection again may enter by the same route.

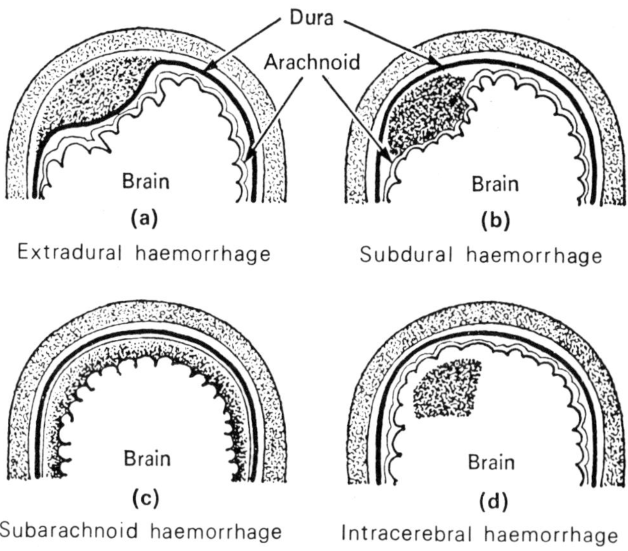

FIG. 5.2 The types of intracranial haemorrhage.

Extradural Haematoma

Injury to the fronto-parietal region may rupture the **middle meningeal artery,** which is an important vessel lying just inside the skull. Bleeding will then occur between the bone and the dura (Fig. 5.2), and an **extradural haematoma** is formed which usually collects and enlarges fairly rapidly. The history in such a case is that the patient has a head injury, is either not knocked unconscious, or recovers consciousness very rapidly, and then within one or two hours becomes increasingly **drowsy,** develops **paralysis** down one side of the body due to pressure of the expanding haematoma on the brain, and dilatation of one pupil, due to stretching of the third nerve. The short period of recovery is very important, for many people are rendered unconscious at the moment of the injury and may remain unconscious with a marked hemiplegia, as a result of severe brain damage, but this is quite different. An extradural haematoma requires an emergency operation. The surgeon will drill a hole in the skull (a **burr-hole** or trephine) over the bruise or fracture site. The clot is sucked out and the patient may recover rapidly, even while this is being done. If it is left alone he will die.

Subdural Haematoma

The fine arteries and veins which run between the arachnoid and dura can also be damaged. In this case a **subdural haematoma** forms (Fig. 5.2). It collects more slowly, so that, though the signs and symptoms are similar to those described, they may be delayed for days or even weeks, and come on much more slowly. Great variations from hour to hour in the degree of **drowsiness** is common and as the clot irritates the cerebral cortex the patient may have **fits.** He also has time to complain of increasing **headache.** In young people the skull almost invariably has to be fractured for this to occur, but in the elderly, whose vessels are more brittle, a subdural haematoma may follow a much milder degree of trauma. Treatment again is by surgical evacuation of the clot.

Traumatic Subarachnoid Bleeding

Tearing the vessels lying between the arachnoid and the pia results in bleeding into the subarachnoid space (Fig. 5.2). This is not uncommon in head injuries. After regaining consciousness, the patient has severe headache for many days with marked stiffness of the neck. This gradually improves, and he neither loses consciousness again nor develops a hemiplegia. Such cases normally recover spontaneously.

Concussion, Contusion, Laceration

The obvious danger from a head injury is damage to the brain itself. This will occur when something such as a bullet pierces the skull and forms a penetrating injury, and may also occur following a depressed fracture. Most head injuries are, however, not penetrating wounds, and the whole brain can be severely 'shaken up' without the skull being fractured. This results in temporary loss of function of the brain cells and temporary loss of consciousness. Sudden acceleration of the skull by the knock-out blow in boxing, or sudden deceleration as a result of a fall on the head, are typical examples of this state, which is called concussion, and need not result in permanent damage to any part of the brain. The patient is 'stunned', 'dazed', or actually unconscious for some minutes, or even hours, and may be confused for several hours afterwards, but recovery occurs with no abnormal signs.

If the injury is more severe, the brain tissue will be bruised. This is called contusion. From this many cells will die, and according to the part of the brain damaged, the signs will vary from mild transient weakness of a limb to prolonged unconsciousness and profound paralysis.

If the brain tissue is actually torn, as is usually the case when there is a compound depressed fracture, then there is likely to be bleeding into and around the tear. A cerebral laceration of this type results in more severe and prolonged unconsciousness and paralysis, coming on at once and leaving permanent scarring and some degree of permanent disability.

Consciousness and the Brain Stem. Why do head injuries cause loss of consciousness?

In the brain stem, in addition to the cranial nerve cells and the fibres passing to and from the spinal cord, there is a network of cells and fibres called the **reticular formation.** It is now known that it is impulses spreading from this to the cerebral cortex that keeps the brain in a state of activity, and the individual in a state of wakefulness. When the reticular formation is damaged, these impulses are cut out with the result that consciousness is lost. Many conditions, e.g. haemorrhages, tumours, can cause this damage, but so also can head injuries, and it is contusion of the brain stem that causes the profound loss of consciousness often seen in which there are no other signs of severe cerebral damage. Some patients with this type of injury lie in coma for weeks, months, sometimes years, constituting good 'copy' for the press, but presenting great nursing problems. In lesser degree consciousness will return after a few days or weeks and recovery can be complete.

The brain stem is closely applied to the **base of the skull,** so that fractures here are particularly likely to be associated with injury to it. There is, however, another important way in which it may receive damage and this is described below.

Tentorial Herniation and the Dilated Pupil

It will be recalled that the tentorium separates the cerebral hemispheres from much of the brain stem and cerebellum, and that the upper brain stem passes through the large opening—the tentorial hiatus (Fig. 3.7). If pressure above the tentorium rises rapidly due to something expanding inside the brain or pressing on it from outside, this hiatus presents the only 'escape valve' (Fig. 5.3). The nearest part of the cerebral hemispheres (part of the temporal lobe called the **uncus**) is then forced, or 'herniated', through the hiatus alongside the stem, squeezing it and damaging its blood supply. This results in haemorrhage or softening in the midbrain and pons, which affects the reticular formation, and so causes rapidly deepening **coma.**

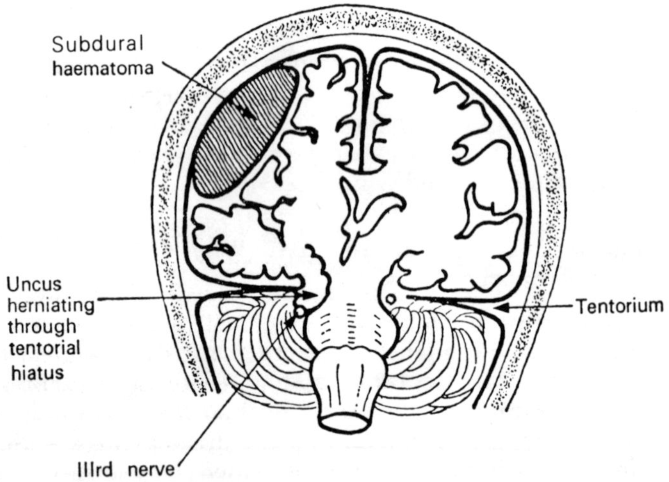

FIG. 5.3 Tentorial herniation, or pressure cone. Note displacement of the IIIrd nerve by the uncus of the temporal lobe as it is 'squeezed' through the tentorial hiatus by the high pressure above.

At the same time the **IIIrd cranial nerve,** which passes near this opening is displaced and stretched by this tentorial herniation. Its automatic fibres are damaged and the **pupil dilates,** first on the side of the herniation, and later on the other side as well.

These signs (increasing coma and a dilating pupil) occur with the late stages of cerebral tumours and abscesses, but they are of particular importance with extradural and subdural haematomas. They are serious omens, and if both pupils are allowed to become dilated and cease to react to light, it may be too late to save the patient, even if the cause is corrected, i.e. the haematoma evacuated, or the tumour removed. Surgical treatment is required before this stage is reached, so the **conscious level** and the **state of the pupils** must be carefully watched in all head injuries, and any change reported at once.

Levels of Consciousness

Drowsiness resembles normal sleep. The patient can easily be wakened and co-operates fully. **Stupor** is a state of unconsciousness in which stimulation produces only restlessness, noisiness and irritability, but no true co-operation. **Coma** is the deepest degree when no response occurs even to the most painful stimulus. Each state merges into the others when unconsciousness is deepening or lightening. In cases of head injury steadily increasing lowering of consciousness is a serious sign for reasons stated above. Failure to regain consciousness that was lost immediately at the time of an accident need not have the same importance, for, though it means cerebral concussion or contusion, it does not necessarily mean increasing bleeding inside the skull.

THE AFTER EFFECTS OF HEAD INJURY

Most patients recover from a head injury without serious ill effects. A few very severe injuries damage the brain stem so badly that consciousness never returns, but modern medical and nursing care may result in survival for many months or years. Others recover consciousness, but the damage to the brain has been so great that they remain mentally abnormal and permanently incapable of looking after themselves. Fortunately these are the small minority, but a much larger number of patients suffer from symptoms which, while not incapacitating, may profoundly alter their way of life afterwards.

Post-traumatic Epilepsy

When the brain is lacerated, a scar forms, which later acts as an **irritating focus** capable of producing **epileptic fits**. Convulsions may occur very shortly (within 24 hours) after a head injury, especially in children. This is due to direct contusion of the brain, or to haemorrhage around it, and need not be of great importance. Some patients, on first getting out of bed after a head injury, have a tendency to lose consciousness easily. These are simple faints and clear up as convalescence progresses. However, some of the more severe head injuries do tend to develop true epileptic convulsions.

This usually happens within the first two years and they need the same type of treatment as in the case of ordinary epilepsy. Epilepsy is most common after a **penetrating wound** through the skull, dura and brain, occurring in 50% of cases, and it is very rare following an injury which has produced only a very short loss of consciousness and no fracture nor intracranial bleeding. Occasionally, when one small part of the brain is damaged, this can be accurately localised by the **electroencephalogram** (see p. 177), and if the patient has very frequent fits it may then be advisable for a surgeon to excise the ragged scar responsible, and replace it by a clean surgical scar which is less likely to cause trouble, but this applies to very few patients.

Post-traumatic Vertigo

Vertigo is a feeling as if the body or the outside world were spinning round. It is often accompanied by **vomiting** and **unsteadiness,** so much so that the patient may fall to the ground, but without losing consciousness. Some degree of vertigo on change of position is common following head injury; it may last for a few days or weeks only, or it may sometimes persist in diminishing degree for many months. It does finally clear up completely.

The Post-concussional Syndrome

Certain patients, following head injury, complain of constant headaches, impairment of memory, increased irritability, intolerance of noise (and therefore of their children), inability to concentrate on reading, hobbies, or even watching television, insomnia, fear of traffic, crowds, or situations similar to those which caused their injury, and above all, inability to work. This rarely follows severe injury and is common following minor injury; it is rare in people of high morale, e.g., jockeys, and Rugby footballers, who frequently suffer such injuries; it is rare if the injury occurs at home, but it is common in factory accidents, road accidents, and accidents which occur under circumstances where some form of financial compensation may be possible. The syndrome is now called **accident neurosis.** It is not due to brain damage and it almost always clears up when the compensation problem is settled, whether in the patient's favour or not. Its exact nature is still a matter of controversy.

SPINAL TRAUMA

Fracture of the bones surrounding the spinal cord is not enough for the cord itself to be damaged. They have to be displaced as well.

The cord may then be crushed, over-stretched, or even completely divided. The result of this is that below the level at which the lesion occurs all the neurones carrying motor impulses are cut off from the muscles they are going to supply, and all the neurones carrying sensation from those parts of the body below the lesion are unable to pass their messages on to the brain. A severe cord lesion will, therefore, cause complete paralysis and complete loss of sensation below a clear cut level. A neck injury produces paralysis of arms, trunk and legs; a thoracic injury, paralysis of the lower part of the trunk and legs; injury to the lumbar spine will probably miss the spinal cord (which, it will be remembered, does not extend below L.1), but it will involve the cauda equina and so produce paralysis of and loss of sensation in the legs and in the bladder.

Immediately after a spinal cord injury at any level there is usually a **flaccid paralysis** of the limbs and complete **retention of urine.** This is due to a state of **'spinal shock'** which usually passes off within three weeks. The flaccidity then changes to **spasticity** if the injury is to the cord itself, owing to damage to the upper motor neurones. If the lesion is in the **cauda equina,** however, the legs remain flaccid, for in this case it is the lower motor neurones that are destroyed. In either case, there is marked loss of skin sensation, the upper level of which corresponds with the level of the damage. In partial lesions of the spinal cord, however, the paralysis and sensory loss show that peculiar distribution known as the Brown–Séquard syndrome, which is described on p. 40.

PERIPHERAL NERVE INJURIES

As most peripheral nerves carry both motor and sensory fibres, injury causes weakness of the muscles they supply and loss of all forms of sensation over the particular area of the skin. Practically any nerve in the body may be injured, but some, because of their position are particularly vulnerable. These are (a) the **ulnar**; this lies very near the surface at the **elbow** and is easily damaged. As a result there is wasting of the hand muscles and loss of sensation over the little finger. (b) the **median**; this is usually involved as it passes through a narrow tunnel at the **wrist,** and it results in wasting of the thumb muscles and loss of sensation over the thumb and first finger. This—the so-called carpal tunnel syndrome—is described on p. 89. (c) the **sciatic**; unhappily, this may easily be injured in the **buttock** by badly placed **injections,** and when this happens there is paralysis of the foot, and loss of sensation over the front and back of the lower leg and foot. (d) the **lateral popliteal**; this may be injured just below the **knees,** perhaps by wearing high boots, or by skin traction for disc lesions, or simply by allowing a thin patient to lie on it. The result is paralysis of dorsiflexion of the foot and loss of sensation between the big toe and the second toe. The other possibilities are too numerous to describe in detail here.

The important thing to remember about all traumatic lesions is that a great deal more nervous tissue is knocked out of action immediately after the injury than is actually destroyed, and astonishing degrees of recovery are possible. It is usually not for many weeks, months, even years that one can confidently say that no further recovery is possible, but by the end of two years, the maximum degree of improvement has usually been reached.

6 *INTRACRANIAL VASCULAR ACCIDENTS*

The **'stroke'** probably remains the best known disorder of the nervous system, and certainly the most feared, yet strictly speaking it is not primarily a neurological disease, but one in which nervous tissue is damaged due to some catastrophe affecting the **blood vessels** carrying the **oxygen** which is so vital for the nerve cells to live. Indeed under normal conditions of body temperature, interruption of all oxygen supply for more than 3–4 minutes results in widespread damage and death to nerve cells, though if body temperature is much reduced (**hypothermia**) they can withstand oxygen lack considerably longer.

When the blood supply to the brain is seriously disturbed spontaneously, i.e. not due to trauma or to surgical ligation of cerebral vessels, we speak of a **cerebrovascular accident,** or **stroke.** There are some forms of vascular accident, however, occurring inside the skull, which do not necessarily damage nervous tissue, and we tend now to group all strokes together as **'intracranial vascular accidents'.** The advances made by special X-ray techniques such as arteriography (see p. 174), and careful pathological studies have considerably altered the traditional views on strokes, and only comparatively recently has this re-thinking become widespread in medical practice.

Characteristics of a Cerebrovascular Accident

(a) The onset is **sudden** or very rapid.
(b) The disability produced is at its **worst at onset** or within a very short period.
(c) If the patient survives the disability tends to **improve,** partially or sometimes even completely.

The Types of Stroke

Strokes can be divided into two major types:

(a) **The ischaemic stroke**, where the supply of blood to a part of the brain suddenly becomes inadequate for the brain cells to function.
(b) **The haemorrhagic stroke,** where a blood vessel ruptures and blood rushes either through the brain tissue destroying it

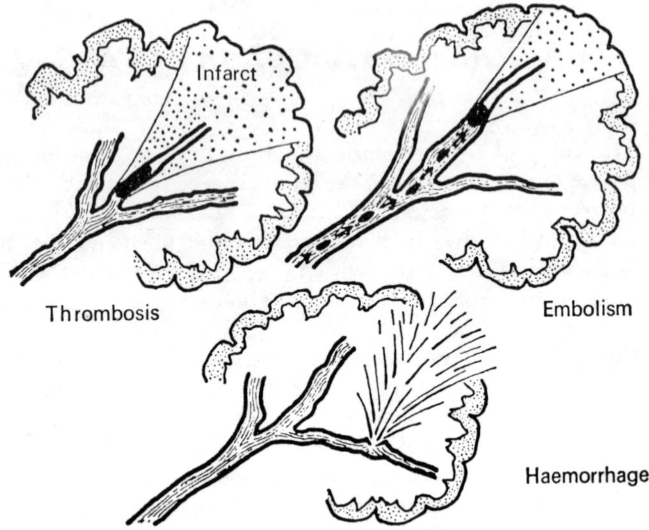

FIG. 6.1 Types of cerebrovascular accident and their effect upon brain tissue.

(**cerebral haemorrhage**), or outside the brain itself into the subarachnoid space (**subarachnoid haemorrhage**). Sometimes both these occur at the same time.

ISCHAEMIC STROKES

The term ischaemic means a shortage of blood supply. There are several ways in which this can occur:

(a) A **blood vessel** in the brain may be **diseased,** the usual disease being **atheroma,** where plaques of hard fatty degenerative nature form on the inner wall of the artery. This impedes blood flow and as a result a **clot** forms, which increases in size, finally blocking the vessel completely. This is then called a **cerebral thrombosis.**

(b) The **clot** may have formed in a vessel **outside** the brain, such as one of the big vessels in the **neck** or **thorax,** or, of course, in the **heart** itself. Pieces of this clot may break off and are carried by the blood stream until they lodge in a vessel too small to allow them to pass further. They then block the vessel and the result is the same as a cerebral thrombosis, but this process is called **cerebral embolism** and the clot responsible is called an **embolus.**

(c) One of the important **blood vessels** supplying the brain (e.g. the carotid or vertebral arteries) may be so diseased that it is markedly **narrowed.** Under normal circumstances enough blood may pass through to nourish the brain, but if something unusual happens, e.g. the patient has a fall in blood pressure on suddenly standing upright, or he twists his neck and 'kinks' an already narrowed artery, there may be a short period in which there is **inadequate flow** through the narrowed vessel. This is usually compensated for by the other blood vessels taking over the duties of the diseased vessel by allowing blood to flow to all the cerebral vessels through connections formed by the **Circle of Willis** (p. 22). However, degenerative disease rarely picks out one vessel alone and it may be that the other vessels are not capable of suddenly supplying more than their territory, and as a result the part of the brain suppled by the original vessel becomes **ischaemic** and a **stroke** results. In this situation, however, there is **no actual blockage** of a vessel and as soon as the circumstances referred to are corrected, **blood flow** is **restored** and so the attack of ischaemia is very transient and the disability rapidly clears up. Indeed such attacks are referred to as **transient ischaemic attacks.**

(d) There is, however, another and perhaps more common cause for transient ischaemic attacks. Once again the **wall** of a blood vessel is **diseased** and on this diseased area small collections of **platelets** stick, **fibrin** or **small clots** are formed and then fragments of these break off, behave as an **embolus,** but instead of blocking an artery inside the brain completely, do so for a few moments only, then break up and pass on through the circulation so that normal blood supply is restored. Indeed if these little emboli pass through the retinal vessels they can be watched by means of an ophthalmoscope and photographed while the patient loses and then recovers his vision.

It is clear, therefore, that all degrees of ischaemic stroke may occur, from the transient ischaemic attack lasting a few minutes, to the total blockage of an important artery.

The Effects of Cerebral Ischaemia

In **complete thrombosis** or **major embolism** of a cerebral vessel the results are the same. A cone-shaped area of brain is rendered short of blood and some of the cells die and never recover; others are temporarily knocked out of action but recover as other vessels take over the task of the one that is blocked. This area is known as a **cerebral infarct,** and the process as **cerebral infarction.**

In **transient ischaemic attacks** the cells are not deprived of blood and oxygen for long enough for them to die, so that they are only temporarily knocked out of action and **blood flow** is **restored** through the temporarily blocked vessel and an infarct does not occur.

However, if in cases of **narrowing** of large vessels resulting in **failure** of **adequate supply,** combined with failure of the other blood vessels to take over the task, then the time the ischaemia lasts may be long enough for an infarct to form, and one is then faced with an area of **cerebral infarction** in which there is **not actual total blockage** of the vessels immediately supplying it. Indeed until the importance of these changes in the balance of blood supply, and the failure of one to substitute for the deficiency of another was fully understood, these areas were something of a mystery. We now realise, however, that the supply of blood to the brain is the result of team work by all the vessels making up the Circle of Willis and if, to use a comparison with football, one of these goes out of action due to disease or injury, a substitute takes over the task, but if that substitute himself is diseased, then it cannot do two jobs at once and naturally concentrates on its own original area, and the other area becomes ischaemic and infarcted.

The Clinical Results of Cerebral Infarction

The **signs** and **symptoms** resulting from cerebral infarction depend entirely on the **area** of the **brain** involved and the proportion of the cells in that area permanently damaged.

In the most general terms the patients will tend to be in the **arteriosclerotic** age group, often, but not necessarily, also **hypertensive**; the infarction will tend to occur when blood flow is **sluggish,** e.g. during sleep, when immobile, after a heavy meal, or when blood pressure suddenly falls, such as when getting out of a warm bed or bath, and assuming an upright position. The loss of function—**paralysis, loss of sensation, loss** of part of the **field of vision, loss of speech,** or all of these—will develop **abruptly** or very rapidly and be at a maximum within a few minutes. This state of **maximum disability** will remain for **hours** or **days,** and then **recovery** will begin and, according to how many cells have been completely destroyed, may be complete in a matter of weeks, or may leave behind some degree of disability, representing part of the original loss of function. Of course, in some cases the infarct is so large that recovery is hardly possible. In other cases, or in transient ischaemic attacks, no true infarct has occurred and recovery is complete in minutes. Headache is not common, loss of consciousness is slight or short lived, and fits do not usually occur.

The exact clinical picture produced is related to the blood vessel whose area of supply is rendered ischaemic. This led to terms such as 'middle cerebral thrombosis', 'posterior inferior cerebellar artery thrombosis' until it was shown by arteriography or autopsy that these vessels in fact were only rarely thrombosed. We now prefer to refer to a **'middle cerebral artery territory infarction'** or ischaemia. The following are the signs which lead one to incriminate the territory of particular arteries.

Middle Cerebral Artery. There is **paralysis** of the **opposite** side of the body, mainly affecting the **face** and **arm,** but if the patient is right handed and the left artery is affected there will also be **loss of speech** (aphasia). The limbs are usually flaccid at first, but as the state of cerebral 'shock' passes off, they become spastic, or may recover completely.

Anterior Cerebral Artery. This is **uncommon** and the **opposite leg** is principally affected.

Posterior Cerebral Artery. Sudden loss of the **opposite half** of the **fields of vision** occurs producing **homonymous hemianopia** (see p. 36).

Basilar Artery. The **brain stem** is gravely disturbed in this case and coma and death often follow. There is gross **disturbance of eye movement,** paralysis of **swallowing,** weakness of all four limbs and often **bilateral blindness.**

Internal Carotid Artery. The symptoms can be so similar to those produced by blockage of the middle cerebral artery that the latter event is often diagnosed in error. This is one of the vessels which comes under suspicion when there are **repeated small strokes,** or transient ischaemic attacks, for it is from plaques of atheroma in the wall of the internal carotid in the neck that **small emboli** may become detached and lodge temporarily in (usually) the middle cerebral artery. Similarly it is in this vessel in the neck that narrowing (**stenosis**) of severe degree may occur, and it is this vessel which may be completely thrombosed in the neck with no signs or symptoms at all because the other vessels, through the Circle of Willis, maintain blood flow to the whole brain, until something happens to disturb their function as well and then it is in the territory of the vessel they are *not* supposed to be supplying that the effects of the ischaemia are felt.

Vertebral Artery. Very much the same remarks apply. One vertebral artery may block without any symptoms, the blood going up the other. If, however, this is also defective, then there are attacks of **vertigo, faintness,** and vague **sensory** disturbances throughout the body, often occurring when the neck is turned or bent. It will be remembered that these two vessels join to form the basilar artery, and it is from inadequate supply to the **brain stem** that symptoms arise.

One striking syndrome of vertebral artery deficiency used to be blamed on thrombosis of the posterior inferior cerebellar artery for it is in its territory that the damage occurs. After an attack of **acute vertigo,** the patient loses **sensation** on **one side** of the **face** and the **opposite side** of the rest of the **body.** This is due to the peculiar arrangement of sensory fibres at this part of the brain stem, and may be followed later by troublesome facial pain.

CEREBRAL ARTERIAL INSUFFICIENCY

It will be seen that quite apart from a full scale thrombosis or major embolism a **relative shortage** of **blood supply** may occur and the term **cerebral arterial insufficiency** has grown up to mean there is not necessarily a complete blockage of an artery, but insufficient blood flow through it to cope with all circumstances. This may also occur as a result of **generalised arteriosclerosis** when all the blood vessels to the brain are diseased and narrowed and there is always an insufficient supply for proper functioning of brain cells. This is not uncommon in **older patients** and results in shrinkage or **atrophy** of the brain. The general term **cerebral arteriosclerosis** is applied to this state in which the early symptoms are gradual **failure of memory,** which at first is mainly for recent events, the memory for early years remaining good. Such symptoms are common in all elderly people, but if the process is unusually severe the patient also becomes **unsteady,** tends to take short, **shuffling steps,** to have attacks of **giddiness,** and to **fall** suddenly. If he suddenly stands up he may actually lose consciousness. Even epileptic attacks may occur, usually in the early hours of the morning. The patient becomes irritable, complains of severe continuous headache, may at times imagine he is being persecuted or neglected, and is very difficult to live with. This sad state may progress to complete loss of mental and physical faculties (**arterio-sclerotic dementia**) and no treatment has been discovered which either prevents or reverses the inevitable deterioration.

CEREBRAL THROMBOSIS AND ORAL CONTRACEPTIVES

Cerebral thrombosis is rare in young women so that when a sharp rise in the number of cases seen by neurologists was seen after about 1963 great concern was felt as it was realised that this was almost entirely occurring in women on 'the Pill'. For several years argument raged over whether this was or was not a true relationship but it is now accepted that there is something between **three** and **six** times the chance of a thrombosis if one of the preparations with **high oestrogen** content is used. This risk has been enormously reduced by the now widespread use of low oestrogen pills, or even those containing no oestrogen at all, though the risk has not been entirely overcome. It is a risk, however, that many would prefer to take than to face the constant fear (and danger) of repeated pregnancies, and in time it seems certain that a preparation having little effect upon the clotting capacity of the blood will be developed. Women who have **hypertension,** a past history of **venous thrombosis,** or a bad history of **migraine,** are in greater danger of cerebral thrombosis, and those in whom the symptoms of migraine change to affect one side of the body only when using the Pill should stop it immediately.

Venous Thrombosis

Thrombi can also form in the veins. This is rare, but occurs occasionally during severe illness, **malnutrition, dehydration,** or following **major operations** or a **confinement.** As the main veins lie on the surface of the brain, patchy areas of the cerebral cortex are involved. The cells are irritated and this causes **recurrent fits,** usually followed by weakness of the parts involved. If the thrombosis spreads in the veins, the fits will also spread to affect more and more of one side of the body and may pass over to the other side as well. This also may very rarely occur as a complication of the use of oral contraceptives.

HAEMORRHAGIC STROKES

In these there is a **rupture** of the wall of a blood vessel and blood rushes (a) into and through the brain, destroying brain tissue by its sheer force. This is what is usually meant by the term **cerebral haemorrhage**; (b) into the substance of the brain forming a large clot—an **intracerebral haematoma**; (c) outside the brain into the subarachnoid space. This is the well-known **subarachnoid haemorrhage**; or (d) any combination of these.

Haemorrhage usually results from (a) weakness in a vessel wall such as is caused by a patch of atheroma; (b) an abnormally **high pressure** inside the vessel (i.e. high blood pressure); or (c) both. It tends to occur in **hypertensive** patients over the age of 55, often during periods of **activity.** The onset is **abrupt,** with bursting **headache, vomiting,** and usually rapid **loss of consciousness.** The breathing is stertorous, there is **profound paralysis** of one side of the body, and the paralysed cheek flaps in and out with each breath. Many die rapidly; others remain unconscious for many days and then die; others recover consciousness and some of the use of their limbs, but are left with **serious disability** and **speech defects.** The prognosis is therefore much worse than for ischaemic strokes.

If an **intracerebral haematoma** is formed this acts as a **space-occupying** lesion, may expand, cause **rising intracranial pressure** and increasing paralysis or deepening coma. Such patients require **surgical operation** and evacuation of the clot may be highly rewarding, providing too much brain tissue has not already been destroyed.

SUBARACHNOID HAEMORRHAGE

This is a special type of intracranial haemorrhage where the **bleeding** occurs into the **cerebro-spinal fluid** in the space between the arachnoid and the pia (Fig. 6.2). Most commonly it is due to a

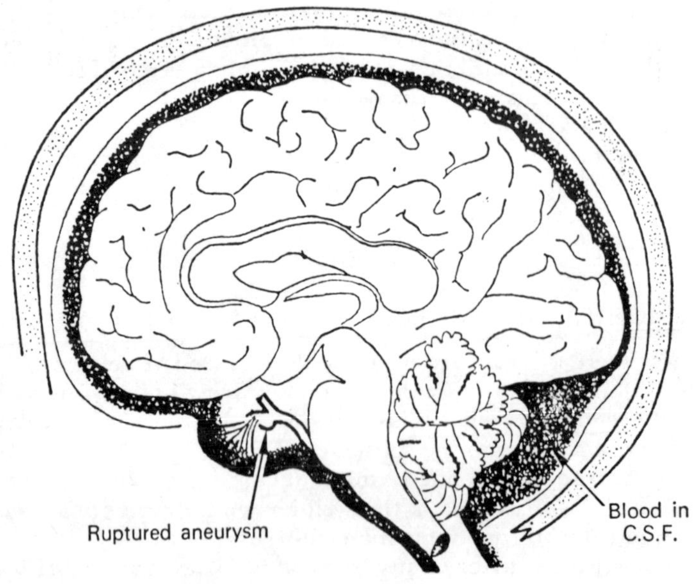

FIG. 6.2 Subarachnoid haemorrhage.

weakness in the wall of a blood vessel at the base of the brain (in the Circle of Willis), but sometimes to rupture of abnormally developed blood vessels which may lie almost anywhere. The two principal causes are **cerebral aneurysms** and **cerebral angiomas.**

Cerebral Aneurysms

The blood is constantly pulsating through the cerebral arteries, and if there is a **weakness** in the wall at the point where they **branch,** a **bulge** will form which is call an **aneurysm** (or a berry aneurysm, because of its appearance) (Fig. 6.3a). It is a very **weak walled sac** and sooner or later it is likely to rupture. The weakness is usually present from birth; intracranial aneurysms are never due to syphilis; but in older patients they may develop owing to **degenerative changes** weakening the vessel wall. They are referred to by the name of the vessel from which they originate, e.g. middle cerebral aneurysm.

The patient can be quite young, with a normal blood pressure and no other vascular disease. He, or she, **suddenly** or very rapidly develops **intense headache** which spreads to the back of the head and down the **neck.** There is repeated **vomiting** and possibly **loss of consciousness.** If not, he develops dislike of light (**photophobia**) and becomes **restless** and irritable. The **neck** becomes **stiff.** Usually there is no paralysis, but if the force of the rupture damages the brain itself, the results can be the same as with an ordinary cerebral haemorrhage. In other cases nearby blood vessels go into **intense spasm,** with the result that cerebral **infarction** and **hemiplegia** occur a few days after the original rupture. In uncomplicated cases the very irritant blood is slowly absorbed from the C.S.F. and after a few days the headache improves, the neck stiffness decreases and the patient may make a complete recovery with no trace of residual disability. These haemorrhages do tend, however, to **recur,** particularly within the first months, and indeed particularly within the first fortnight, and unless the aneurysm can be treated there is quite a high chance of further ruptures proving fatal.

Aneurysms sometimes press on a nearby cranial nerve before they rupture. **The IIIrd nerve** is particularly involved, so that **ptosis** and **paralysis of eye movement** usually need to be investigated by arteriography, unless the patient is too old.

Cerebral Angioma

Sometimes during development blood vessels are formed in an abnormal manner; **arteries** connect directly with **veins** instead of through capillaries; or masses of abnormal capillaries join together. Such abnormal formations are called **vascular anomalies.** An **angioma,** or an **arterio-venous aneurysm** (Fig. 6.3b) is a mass of **abnormal arteries, capillaries** and **veins,** which have abnormally fragile walls, and if lying inside the head are liable to **rupture** and produce subarachnoid haemorrhage. They are usually on or near the

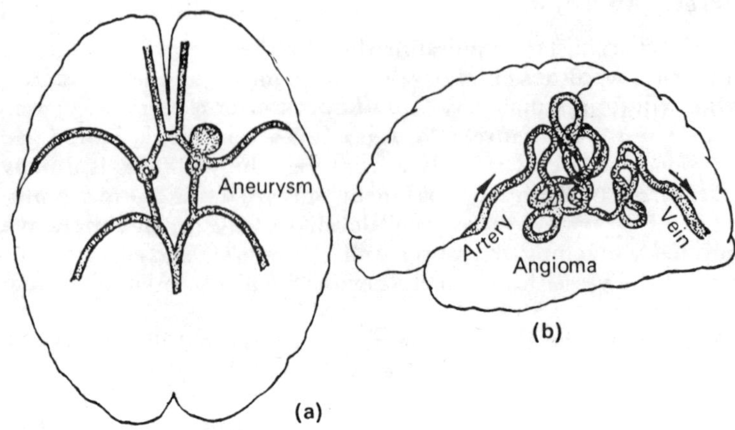

FIG. 6.3 Types of vascular anomaly. (a) An aneurysm on the Circle of Willis; (b) an angioma (or arterio-venous malformation) on the surface of the brain.

cerebral **cortex,** act as an irritant, and tend to produce **fits,** a symptom which does not occur with berry aneurysms. The blood rushes through these widened vessels and it is often possible to hear a pulsating noise by listening to the head with a stethoscope. This is called an **intracranial bruit** and is almost diagnostic of an angioma in an adult.

Differentiating between Thrombosis and Haemorrhage

Arteriography and modern techniques of pathology have shown that it is often very difficult for a clinician to be certain whether he is dealing with a massive cerebral thrombosis (which may mimic a haemorrhage) or a small haemorrhage (which may resemble in every respect a cerebral thrombosis). This is why neurologists always wish to investigate carefully those patients in whom accurate diagnosis might lead to beneficial treatment, and why they are reluctant to prescribe anticoagulants without being sure of what has happened (see below).

The Treatment of Intracranial Vascular Catastrophes

Treatment is far from satisfactory. It can be considered under two headings; (a) the management of the patient following catastrophe and (b) the prevention of further similar episodes. When the stroke occurs the damage to the brain is done in a matter of seconds and nothing can alter its course at that moment. It is any resultant coma and paralysis that require treatment and these nursing problems are described in Chapter 21.

Prevention of Further Catastrophes

There is little that can be done to stop the thrombosis of small brain vessels. **Anticoagulants** are **dangerous** because by reducing the clotting tendency of the blood they may convert a small infarct into a massive haemorrhage. If, however, it has been shown that the main thrombus lies in one of the **large vessels** in the **neck,** from which **small emboli** are being thrown off into the intracranial vessels, then **prolonged** treatment by anticoagulants is often helpful, but it must be shown that this is the case because nothing could be more dangerous than to give anticoagulants if it were in fact a small haemorrhage that had occurred. Therefore, when symptoms suggest a **carotid** artery lesion (e.g. **transient ischaemic** episodes, **recurrent small strokes), arteriography** is normally carried out if the patient is not too old. If the carotid artery is found not to be completely blocked, but **stenosed** (markedly narrowed) it may be possible for a surgeon to cut out the narrowed area, and join the ends of the vessel together again, or put in a **vessel graft,** aiming to restore the full flow of blood.

In young people, **emboli** often come from a **diseased heart,** though even this is uncommon unless the patient is in atrial fibrillation, or the heart is affected by bacterial endocarditis. The heart condition must be corrected as far as is possible, but anticoagulants are again indicated here.

It is possible to **reduce** the **clotting** tendency less drastically by using regular dosage of **aspirin,** and this somewhat unexciting form of treatment has reduced recurrent micro-emboli in many patients.

In cases with cerebral **haemorrhage** due to **hypertension** attempts should be made to **lower** the **blood pressure.** Unless a definite haematoma has formed it is hardly ever of value to try to operate on a hypertensive cerebral haemorrhage. **Subarachnoid haemorrhage,** however, is a different matter altogether.

The Medical Treatment of Subarachnoid Haemorrhage

At first the patient should be allowed to lie in the position most comfortable to him until the headache has subsided. If the diagnosis is suspected a **lumbar puncture** will probably be carried out for confirmation by demonstrating **blood** in the C.S.F. For the first two days after the haemorrhage any **unnecessary movement** should be **avoided,** and the patient should not, if possible, be moved from hospital to hospital, ward to ward, or bed to bed. Analgesics should be given as required and vomiting reduced by Largactil. The patient should be kept strictly in bed for 4-5 weeks, and have a convalescence of a further 3-4 weeks. There is little evidence that any special precautions after this stage reduces the risk of a further haemorrhage, though avoidance of excessive straining (e.g. through constipation) or repeated jolting of the head (e.g. playing soccer) would be wise. Nowadays most cases are referred for surgery, but the stage at which this done varies according to the preference of the surgeon and the condition of the patient.

The Surgical Treatment of Vascular Anomalies

The **prognosis** of subarachnoid haemorrhage has been **greatly improved** by advances in **neurosurgery. Angiography** should normally be carried out as soon as possible to show whether there is an **aneurysm** or **angioma** present, where it is and how big it is. If the bulge of an aneurysm has a **clear cut neck,** the surgeon can place a **clip** across this; if not, he may wrap **muscle** and **gauze** around it to 'splint' it; or he may **tie** the **parent vessel** on either side of the aneurysm. The aim is to take this dangerous weak point out of the circulation. **Angiomas** on the surface of the brain look terrifying, but providing that the main artery feeding them can be clipped, they can often be removed without great difficulty. In either case, if surgery is successful, the **prognosis** is **excellent** and it relieves the patient from the constant fear of a further haemorrhage, which might possibly be fatal (see p. 164).

OTHER DISEASE OF THE BLOOD VESSELS

Polyarteritis Nodosa. This is a rare **inflammatory,** or possibly **allergic,** disease of arteries, which affects all vessels, including those in the brain, spinal cord and peripheral nerves. Repeated vascular catastrophes occur in widely different parts of the nervous system, and the small vessels supplying different **peripheral nerves** become blocked, so that the nerves become paralysed. It is one of the so-called **collagen diseases,** which include **disseminated lupus erythematosus,** another disease giving a similar clinical picture. The blood sedimentation rate is very high, the serum proteins abnormal, and the diagnosis may be confirmed by muscle biopsy.

Temporal Arteritis. This is an **inflammation** of the walls of the arteries of the scalp. It is limited to **elderly** people. The vessels outside the skull become so inflamed and so intensely painful and tender, that the patient cannot bear to wear a hat, or touch the head, or rest it on a pillow. The condition will subside eventually, but unfortunately the ophthalmic artery is often affected and sudden blindness on both sides may occur.

The treatment of these two conditions has been greatly improved by the use of **A.C.T.H.** and **cortisone,** which can produce complete cure, especially in the case of temporal arteritis.

SPINAL VASCULAR DISEASE

Thrombosis or rupture of the spinal arteries is very rare. If these occur it is usually as a complication of some other disease, pressure on the arteries (by a prolapsed disc or a spinal tumour) producing thrombosis; or anomalies of the vessels (angiomas) producing haemorrhage. If a diagnosis of spontaneous spinal thrombosis is made, it is almost always wrong.

7 *INFECTION AND INFLAMMATION OF THE NERVOUS SYSTEM*

The nervous system and its coverings can be infected by the same bacteria and viruses which affect other organs of the body, and the illnesses so caused may be **acute,** as in the case of poliomyelitis; **subacute** (some forms of encephalitis); or long drawn out and **chronic,** as in neurosyphilis.

The result of infection is, at first, inflammation of tissue. Inflammation of the meninges (usually the pia and arachnoid) is called **meningitis;** of the brain, **encephalitis**; and of the spinal cord, **myelitis.** The diagnosis of 'meningism' or 'meningismus' is not often made these days, except in children. It then refers to symptoms and signs suggestive of meningitis but the site of the infection lies elsewhere in the body. These terms are still used however to indicate signs of *irritation* of the meninges without necessarily meaning that they are *directly infected.* **Neuritis** should mean inflammation of a peripheral nerve, and **polyneuritis** of many nerves. However it is only rarely that nerves are directly infected, and these terms are discussed on page 114. If the nerve root is thought to be inflamed, the term **radiculitis** is used.

MENINGITIS

There are three main types of meningitis (a) **pyogenic,** i.e. caused by pus-forming bacteria, the commonest being meningococci, pneumococci and the influenza bacillus; (b) **tuberculous,** caused by the tubercle bacillus; and (c) **viral,** caused by a number of different viruses, some of which are known (e.g. polio virus, mumps virus), others being presumed, but not proved, to be the cause.

The Symptoms of Meningeal Infection

There are certain features which occur in all the types of meningitis. The illness starts with a few days of pyrexia, a vague influenza-like state, a cold or sore throat. This is followed by a rapidly developing **headache,** which spreads backwards to give pain in the neck and back. It is accompanied by **vomiting, photophobia,** and the patient then becomes drowsy, but restless and irritable, and shows the vital sign of meningeal irritation, no matter what cause—neck stiffness or **neck rigidity.** This is demonstrated by attempting unsuccessfully to bend the head forwards so as to bring the chin on to the chest (Fig. 7.1a). In addition, **Kernig's sign** is positive. To test for this, the hip is first flexed, and then an attempt is made to straighten the knee (Fig. 7.1b). If the sign is positive, the movement is restricted and very painful to the patient.

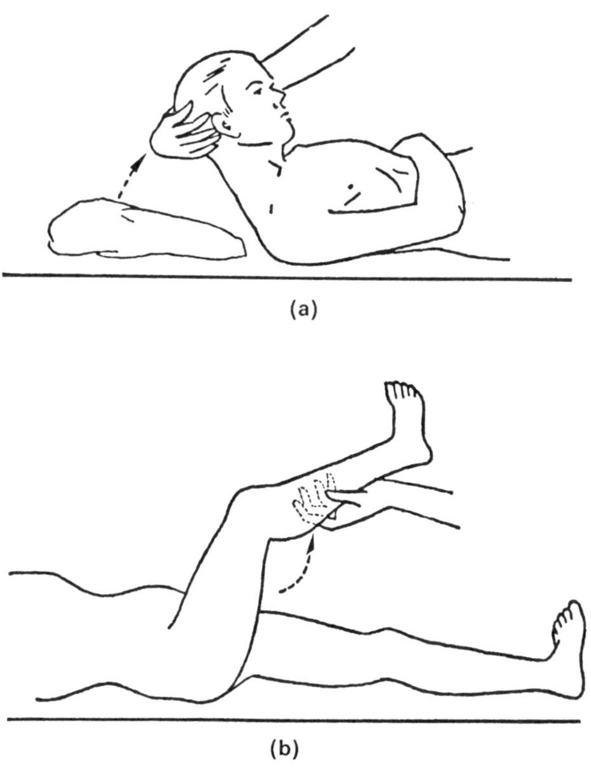

FIG. 7.1 Tests for meningeal irritation or meningitis. (a) Testing for neck rigidity; (b) testing for Kernig's sign.

In infants the spasm of the neck muscles may be so great that the neck is bent backwards **(neck retraction),** or the whole body arched **(opisthotonos).** Neck rigidity or retraction *without* Kernig's sign may be present when high pressure within the skull has thrust the cerebellar tonsils down through the foramen magnum forming a pressure cone, see p. 171.

Pyogenic Meningitis

Meningococcal meningitis is spread by nasopharyngeal infection, and may occur in epidemics. Pneumococcal meningitis often follows pneumonia, or when a fracture of the skull has passed through the nasal air sinuses (see p. 43). Influenzal meningitis especially appears in infants. The symptoms and signs are as described above. The diagnosis is confirmed by doing a lumbar puncture, when the C.S.F. pressure will be raised, the fluid cloudy, or milky, and containing thousands of polymorphonuclear leucocytes (i.e. pus cells), and a much reduced sugar. Some of the C.S.F. is placed on a slide and stained to try to find the responsible organism, and further specimens are placed on culture plates with various drugs to find to which it is most sensitive (i.e. which prevents it from growing).

These examinations take time, and treatment must be started at once, so the patients are immediately put on penicillin and sulphonamides, and, in the case of suspected pneumococcal infection, diluted penicillin may also be given directly into the C.S.F. by repeated lumbar punctures. When the organism has been identified and its sensitivity decided the antibiotic may have to be changed, but most cases of these formerly fatal diseases can now be cured.

Tuberculous Meningitis

The onset of this disease is much less acute. The patient may have been vaguely unwell for weeks, with gradually increasing headache and listlessness. He may, of course, be known to have tuberculosis elsewhere, but this is not common. Finally, the same symptoms and signs as in other cases of meningitis develop, but the C.S.F. shows fewer cells, polymorphs and lymphocytes are present in about equal numbers, and both sugar and chlorides are very low.

This disease used to be invariably fatal, but now the majority can be saved by a prolonged course of streptomycin injections, together with iso-nicotinic acid hydrazide (I.N.A.H.), and para-aminosalicylic acid (P.A.S.) by mouth. Streptomycin used also to be given directly into the C.S.F. by daily lumbar puncture and this may still be necessary in some adults, but the majority of children respond to the intramuscular injections alone. This is, of course, a great blessing, to both patient and medical attendants. Treatment has to be given for at least three months.

Viral Meningitis

The onset and the symptoms are similar to the pyogenic forms, but are usually less severe, and the diagnosis is suspected when the

C.S.F. is found to be clear and to contain mainly lymphocytes, while the sugar and chlorides are normal. As yet, no drug definitely affects these infections, but fortunately the patient usually makes a spontaneous recovery. Gradually more viruses (E.C.H.O., coxsackie) are being identified as responsible but often the diagnosis is only a presumptive one.

ENCEPHALITIS

Inflammation of the brain is called encephalitis, and if the meninges are involved at the same time we speak of **meningo-encephalitis**. As with meningitis, the infection may be due to pyogenic bacteria, or to viruses, or in some countries to various forms of parasite acquired from animals.

General Features of Encephalitis

The symptoms consist of moderate **headache, vomiting, confusion, delirium,** increasing **drowsiness** which passes into coma, and epileptic **fits.** The fits may be frequent and spread to involve increasing areas of the body as the cerebral inflammation extends. Unless the meninges are also infected there is relatively little neck stiffness, Kernig's sign is negative, and the C.S.F. may be under normal pressure and show a moderate rise in lymphocytes only, without any other special features. The seriousness of the disease depends upon which organisms are responsible. Encephalitis due to pyogenic bacteria will kill the patient unless treated, whereas a patient with viral encephalitis may recover without serious after effects. Even this is uncertain, however, and some patients show changes in personality, with a tendency towards outbursts of temper, fits, and difficulty in learning, so that their whole future is disrupted.

Pyogenic Encephalitis

Bacterial infection can spread directly into the brain from the **nasal sinuses,** or from **infected ears,** or it may be carried by the blood from **infected lungs** (e.g. in cases of bronchiectasis). In **congenital heart disease** with communication between the right and left sides of the heart, infection can be more easily carried to the brain from areas such as **infected teeth,** and of course, infected pieces of thrombus can spread from **diseased heart valves** in bacterial endocarditis. Part of the brain first becomes swollen (oedematous), and then the inflamed area liquefies and white blood cells pour in until a collection of pure pus is formed. This is a **cerebral abscess**

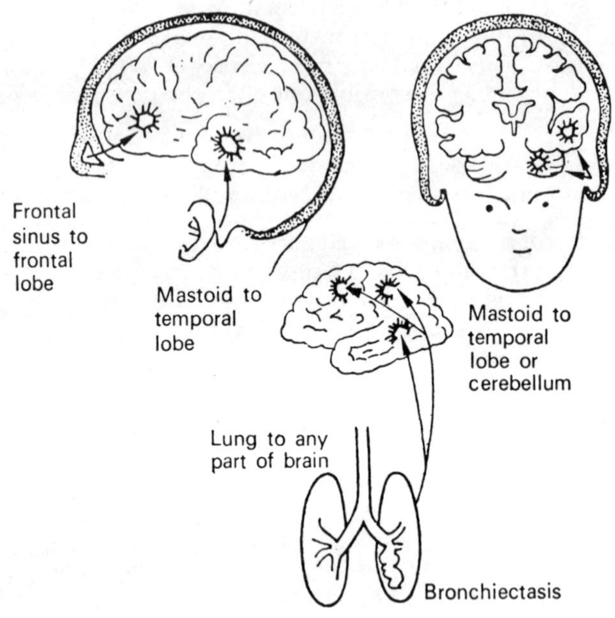

FIG. 7.2 The origins of cerebral abscesses and the common sites for them to occur.

(Fig. 7.2). Abscesses most commonly develop in the frontal or temporal lobes. The brain tries to form a protective fibrous barrier, which is called a **capsule** around this abscess, and the older the abscess the thicker the capsule. At first the symptoms are the same as for encephalitis generally, but they are more severe and acute, and paralysis of limbs is common. As the abscess enlarges it produces signs similar to those of a tumour (see p. 79).

Cerebral abscesses are now treated surgically. Their position can be located by brain scanning and by X-rays (especially arteriography), a burr-hole is made in the skull and a needle is passed into the centre of the abscess. Pus is withdrawn, slides and cultures prepared and an antibiotic is introduced, together with a substance opaque to X-rays. Organisms are not always grown, but if they are, their sensitivity is tested, for some other antibiotics may be more suitable. Aspiration and replacement by the antibiotic will be carried out fairly frequently at first, while the size of the abscess is watched on repeated X-rays. This is possible because the opaque material is taken up by the capsule and outlines the abscess. It will gradually shrink and eventually may be excised completely.

Viral Encephalitis

In recent years we have seen considerable advances in the diagnosis and treatment of some of these conditions. It was once very rare to isolate a virus and more help was obtained from showing a rise in the level of antibodies in the blood, from which a diagnosis was presumed. However, new techniques and the use of the electron microscope have altered the situation considerably.

By these means **herpes simplex encephalitis** has become one of the most common varieties to be recognised. The clinical picture resembles that of cerebral abscess in many ways. Brain scanning shows abnormal uptake in the temporal lobes; arteriography shows displacement, deformity and excess of blood vessels in these areas and, as it is essential to make the diagnosis accurately and quickly when it is suspected, a burr-hole is made, a small portion of brain tissue is taken (which also enables an abscess to be excluded) and special **fluorescent stains** for **herpes antibodies** are carried out while the virus itself can be recognised under the **electron microscope.** The answer can be given in a few hours; the matter is one of great urgency, for by the use of steroids such as dexamethazone, combined possibly with anti-viral drugs such as cytarabine, an otherwise fatal outcome may be prevented. This unhappily does not mean that all patients make complete recovery—the residual mental and physical disability may be severe. For this reason the relative value of different methods of treatment is still very much under review.

Encephalitis Lethargica

Between 1918 and 1925 a great epidemic of encephalitis lethargica or **sleeping sickness** occurred in Europe. It was presumably of virus origin though the virus was never found. It may have been a variety of the influenza virus and though now very rare, isolated examples of a very similar clinical picture may be seen from time to time. The **brain stem** was particularly affected, so that as well as the general symptoms, there was paralysis of eye movement, and the patients were drowsy by day and wakeful at night. The face became rigid, and there was considerable personality disturbance. Recovery usually occurred but there was an important after-effect—a type of Parkinsonism (**post-encephalitic Parkinsonism,** see p. 108) which did not necessarily appear for many years.

The Subacute Forms of Encephalitis

There are a number of rare, gradually developing inflammations of the brain which are almost confined to children, are of unknown origin, and usually start by slowly progressive **mental deterioration,** followed by **fits, tremulousness, ataxia** and finally extreme spasticity and **rigidity.** Subacute sclerosing panencephalitis or inclusion body encephalitis is the best known of this group, in which these symptoms are accompanied by attacks of drooping of the head and limbs followed by tremor, and the electroencephalogram gives an almost diagnostic abnormality. Brain biopsy may again be necessary to make certain of the diagnosis, for so far there is no treatment which checks this almost certainly fatal, but prolonged, illness. There is now very strong evidence that this disease may be a chronic form of measles infection.

Another rare encephalitis, almost invariably fatal and affecting adults and presenting as a **progressive dementia** with **tremors** and **characteristic E.E.G.** picture is named after those who first described it as the **Jakob-Creuzfeld disease.** This is an important disease, because it has been possible to transmit it to experimental animals though it takes a long time to show its effects. It is thought to be due to one of what are now known as the **'slow' viruses,** which are thought to be responsible for several hitherto unexplained progressive neurological disorders.

SPINAL INFECTIONS

Pyogenic Infections

Pyogenic infections of the spinal cord itself are rare. An abscess may form in the fat outside the meninges (extradural spinal abscess) producing pain and tenderness in the back and a rapidly developing paralysis of the legs. This usually follows infected skin lesions, or (happily rarely) epidural anaesthesia for childbirth. If an abscess has formed it is drained surgically but in the earliest stage of infection of the epidural space antibiotic therapy may be sufficient.

Tuberculous Infections

Tuberculous infections may cause collapse of a vertebra (Pott's disease), or a paravertebral tuberculous abscess. Either can cause cord compression and paraplegia, but these are usually treated by immobilisation and streptomycin.

Poliomyelitis

Acute anterior poliomyelitis, to give its full name, is a better term than infantile paralysis, for nowadays quite 50% of patients are adults. The poliomyelitis virus has been isolated and it produces its effects by attacking the **motor cells** in the **anterior horns** of the spinal cord. In the more severe cases the motor cells in the medulla and the brain stem are also affected and the process is then called **polioencephalitis.** A few cases occur each year, but epidemics may develop from time to time.

The virus enters the blood stream through the nasopharynx and intestinal tract, and invades the meninges first, causing a **lymphocytic meningitis.** The onset is acute with pyrexia, headache, vomiting, stiffness of the neck and pain in the back and limbs. This stage lasts 2-4 days and may subside completely. This is what is known as **non-paralytic poliomyelitis** and in any epidemic cases of this type greatly exceed those which develop any paralysis. They are, however, the main source of spread of the infection, but except during an epidemic, they are difficult to distinguish from any other viral meningitis.

In a few cases, after this stage there is about 48 hours interval, and then the **paralytic stage** begins, with pain and extreme tenderness of various muscles. The muscles rapidly become weak or even totally paralysed. The danger rises when the respiratory muscles, diaphragm and intercostals are affected, and, in polioencephalitis, the muscles of the throat, for the patient is unable to swallow, cough, or breathe properly. It was for these patients that the 'iron lung' was developed, now largely replaced by other forms of artificial respiration.

When the acute stage has settled down, many muscles recover completely, but others may waste, at times almost completely. Even in these a great deal of function may be restored by physiotherapy and rehabilitation, but some muscles remain permanently withered. If the patient is a small child the affected limb may not grow as quickly as the others.

The poliomyelitis **virus** can be detected in the **faeces** of the patients with the non-paralytic variety, and in the early stages of the paralytic disease. Tests for **antibodies** can also be carried out in the blood. This makes it possible to confirm the diagnosis in a dubious case, and to detect those who might be carriers.

Treatment

The pre- or non-paralytic stage requires no treatment other than rest and analgesics for the headache. **Rest,** however, is of greatest importance if the disease is suspected, for physical exercise during this stage greatly increases the chances of paralysis developing.

Doctors have no wonder drug to treat the acute stage of the paralysis, and a great responsibility rests on the nurse. From the very beginning it must be assumed that the patient is going to make a good recovery. The **limbs** must, therefore, be carefully supported in positions which will avoid overstretching of the muscles. The **joints** must be protected. Pain and **spasms** in the muscles can be eased by applying **hot packs,** but movement, e.g. for the treatment of pressure areas, should be avoided for several days. The **respiration** and **pulse** rate must be watched carefully for respiratory embarrassment may develop rapidly. When the pain subsides each joint must be moved by the nurse through its full range twice each day to avoid its becoming 'stuck' in one position, and care of pressure points, urine and bowels are as important as in coma and paraplegia (pp. 179–185).

Most patients know about the **'iron lung'.** It is an ugly term and rather frightening. The original mechanical respirators have been greatly improved allowing nursing to be carried out with much greater ease. They are divided into upper and lower halves, hinged at one end so that they can be opened widely and the process of first placing the patient in is much easier than formerly. Many patients with respiratory paralysis also develop difficulty in swallowing. This is dangerous for saliva, fluids and sputum may be aspirated into the lungs. The foot of the respirator must be well **elevated,** the patient nursed on his face and the head turned to one side, for secretions will then drain away from the trachea and can be sucked out. In such cases a tracheostomy will be performed making it possible to keep the airway clear by sucking out the trachea efficiently. In fact the use of controlled respiration by connecting a pump to the tracheostomy tube and inflating the lungs by positive pressure has largely replaced the use of the box-type respirators, and as the patient is not encased nursing is made infinitely easier. A team of experts is required for this type of work demanding the co-operation of doctors, nurses and physiotherapists. For this reason most cases are now transferred to special respiration units.

As the patient recovers, artificial respiration will be stopped for increasing periods each day. When finally able to breathe unaided, he may nevertheless need artificial help during periods of respiratory infection. A few patients never regain their own powers of respiration.

Rehabilitation of severely paralysed patient requires the team work of physiotherapists, surgeons, and instrument makers. Recovery of power usually continues for up to two years, after which the condition is static, but the patients are taught to overcome their disability and there are now numerous ingenious appliances available to help a paralysed limb to carry out almost normal activity.

Prevention. Modern **immunisation** campaigns have transformed the picture in the world as a whole, the paralytic disease now being uncommon in immunised individuals, though so far the incidence of *non*-paralytic poliomyelitis does not seem to have been greatly affected.

CHRONIC INFLAMMATORY DISEASE

Syphilis

Syphilitic infection of the nervous system does not appear for many years after the original infection. The organism, a spirochaete, *Treponema pallidum,* causes chronic inflammation of the nervous tissue and its coverings and produces three main diseases:—**meningo-vascular syphilis, tabes dorsalis,** and **general paralysis of the insane** (**G.P.I.**). Once common in every neurological ward, these diseases have become very rare as a result of the successful early treatment of syphilis. They do still occur however, especially in countries where effective early treatment may not be easily available, and one is in danger of not making the diagnosis unless constantly on the alert. Our more 'permissive' society has resulted in an increase of venereal disease in young people so that the danger of neurosyphilis may become greater in years ahead.

Meningo-vascular Syphilis

This infection involves the meninges, causing them to be inflamed and thickened, and also the blood vessels supplying the brain and cord, thickening their walls and narrowing their lumen. Episodes of thrombosis therefore occur, causing sudden paralysis of one of the cranial nerves, or of a limb. The C.S.F. shows a slightly raised lymphocyte count and the **blood W.R.** will usually be **positive,** though the C.S.F. W.R. may be negative. The clinical picture can be so varied, so many parts of the nervous system can be involved, and so many other diseases imitated, that it is wise to do a W.R. routinely in all neurological problems.

Tabes Dorsalis

Here the **sensory roots** are affected as they enter the spinal cord, and there is degeneration of the fibres running up in the posterior (dorsal) columns (tabes = wasting). The root irritation causes **'lightning' pains,** which are sudden bursts of needle-like pains in the shins, calves, and arms; and **'girdle pains'** which are more prolonged sensations resembling a constricting band around the trunk. The posterior column lesion causes **loss of position sense** so that the patient becomes ataxic and walks with legs wide apart with a stamping gait, and becomes almost helpless in the dark. The degeneration of sensory fibres upsets the reflex arc (p. 26) so that the **tendon reflexes** are **absent,** and disturbs sensation in the bladder, so that there is no desire to pass urine, there is overfilling, and **overflow incontinence.** Patchy areas of loss of sensation occur on the skin and these may result in **ulcers** on the feet. Gross destructive changes take place in the knees and other joints, but owing to loss of sensory fibres these changes are painless. The resulting disorganised joints are called **Charcot's joints.** Perhaps the most characteristic sign of neurosyphilis is in the eyes—the so-called **Argyll Robertson pupil.** This is a small irregular pupil, which does not react to light, but does constrict on looking at a near object. The C.S.F. in the active disease shows a raised lymphocyte count, and a tabetic (luetic) Lange curve (this is explained on p. 193). The W.R. may be negative, both in the blood (40%) and in the C.S.F. (20%), but in patients who have been given penicillin at some time in the past, the W.R. may even more frequently be negative. More complex tests then have to be done to show the presence of antibodies to the organisms causing syphilis (e.g. **treponema immobilisation** and **fluorescent antibody** tests) which may be positive when the W.R. is negative.

General Paralysis of the Insane (G.P.I.)

It is the nerve cells of the brain that are involved in this type of neurosyphilis. Many of them die and the brain atrophies, or shrinks. The symptoms are those of slow **mental deterioration** accompanied sometimes by the so-called **grandiose delusions,** in which the patient imagines himself rich, famous, or having done great deeds. There are often **fits,** and signs of upper motor neurone disease develop with spasticity, exaggerated reflexes and extensor plantars. Argyll Robertson pupils are common, and the **W.R.** is **positive** in **100%** of untreated cases in the C.S.F., the Lange curve (p. 193) being of paretic type.

Many patients have features of both tabes and G.P.I., when the condition is known as **tabo-paresis** and this is more common now than formerly. Occasionally children of syphilitic parents may develop juvenile G.P.I. or tabes.

Treatment of Neurosyphilis

Treatment used to be arduous and to the modern practitioner must seem strange. It ranged from long courses of injections of arsenic and bismuth, or rubbing mercurial ointments into the skin, to infecting the G.P.I. patients with malaria. Now, however, **penicillin** is the treatment of choice. A total of 20 000 000 units should be given in divided doses over about 10–12 days. This usually cures meningovascular syphilis, and greatly improves the situation in G.P.I., but is often disappointing in tabes. Even in tabes it is still simpler, less dangerous, and no less effective than the older methods. The courses have to be repeated at 3- or 6-monthly intervals until all signs of activity have cleared up. The common use of penicillin for other reasons has made diagnosis of neurosyphilis harder, and the classical clinical pictures are much less common.

Tuberculosis

Tuberculous meningitis has already been described, but occasionally chronic tuberculous lesions form in the brain and meninges. These consist of tumour-like masses of cells (tuberculoma) in the centre of which are tubercle bacilli, and they may behave like a tumour, or they may rupture into the meninges and cause a tuberculous meningitis. To distinguish them from tumours, they are called **granulomas.** They are difficult to diagnose, and have to be investigated as a tumour, but once the diagnosis is made they are treated by **streptomycin.** Sometimes it is necessary to biopsy a suspected tuberculoma in order to confirm the diagnosis. If this is to be done streptomycin is started beforehand to prevent spread of infection.

Sarcoidosis

In this curious condition granulomas develop which are similar to tuberculomas, but do not contain tubercle bacilli. Their origin is uncertain. They form in the brain, meninges, around the peripheral nerves, and in glands throughout the body, and the condition is usually diagnosed by **biopsy** of one of these **glands.** Treatment is by **cortisone.**

Leprosy

The leprosy bacillus causes the peripheral nerves to become thickened so that they can be both seen and felt. Sensation is lost in those parts of the body supplied by these nerves, and **trophic changes** eventually occur. As a result areas of skin and bone slough off, causing **mutilation** of the hands, feet and face. Most patients diagnosed in this country have come from India or the Middle East. Contrary to popular belief it is only a slightly infectious disease, and modern treatment with sulphones offers a considerable hope of cure.

OTHER INFECTIONS INVOLVING NERVOUS TISSUE

Herpes Zoster

The zoster virus invades the **ganglia** which lie on the posterior roots of the spinal nerves and on the trigeminal nerve. The illness starts with severe **pain** in the distribution of the nerve root, often around the trunk, or above the eyes in the case of **ophthalmic herpes** which particularly affects the elderly. At first red patches appear on the skin. These change into **vesicles,** which run together and then crust over and heal, leaving pale depressed scars like those after chicken-pox. In fact there is a relationship between the virus of herpes zoster and that of chicken-pox. In elderly patients the pain may persist in the affected area for many years and becomes the major obsession of their lives. No treatment so far discovered has been consistently helpful. In **geniculate herpes** the vesicles develop on the ear, and there is often facial paralysis and deafness.

Parasitic Infections

Various parasites may affect the nervous system, but they are rare in this country. **Tapeworms** have an intermediate or larval form, which usually develops in some other animal. The human tapeworm *Taenia solium* can at times develop its larval stage not, as normally, in the pig, but in the human muscle and brain. These larvae are called **cysticerci** and the condition, **cysticercosis.** The muscle cysts are harmless, but they calcify and can be seen in X-rays of the thighs and pelvis. Those in the brain cause epilepsy and sometimes mental changes. The patients have usually contracted the disease in the Far East, South America, or Eastern Europe.

Another parasite, *Trichinella spiralis,* affects humans if they eat uncooked sausage meat. It usually develops in the muscles and the eyelids, but it can produce a serious encephalitis. The condition is called **trichiniasis,** and it is common in America among Negro children.

Hydatid disease—cysts formed by the parasite *Echinococcus*—is very rare, but may develop in the brain, skull, or meninges and behaves like a cerebral tumour. This is common in Australia and the Middle East, and is seen in South and Mid-Wales and some eastern areas of England, essentially in sheep-rearing communities.

Leptospirosis is caused by organisms carried by rats and dogs. The dog variety, *Leptospira canicola,* causes a high fever, meningitis, and inflammation of the eyes, which is known as **canicola fever.**

Suppression of Immunity

A relatively recent problem of infection has arisen from the widespread use of **immuno-suppressive drugs,** used frequently after **transplant** operations, for instance, to try and prevent **'rejection'**; also in certain diseases such as Hodgkin's disease, and of course in many other conditions for which steroids (cortisone, prednisolone) are given. These allow certain viruses to affect the nervous system which normally are resisted by immunity. An **encephalitic illness** may follow high dosage of these preparations, and sometimes it is this rather than the original disease which kills the patient.

8 *TUMOURS*

Tumours (neoplasms) affecting the nervous system are said to be **primary** if they grow from cells of the nervous system itself; or **secondary** (metastases) if they are carried to the nervous system by the blood from a primary tumour elsewhere, e.g. bronchus, or breasts. They can be **extrinsic,** which means they grow outside the brain or spinal cord; or **intrinsic,** growing within the substance of the nervous tissue. Most extrinsic tumours are benign growing slowly and compressing nervous tissue, but remaining quite separate from it. They do not spread elsewhere. Most intrinsic tumours are malignant, growing more quickly and destroying nervous tissue by spreading all through it so that one cannot tell where tumour ends and normal tissue begins. Metastases to other parts of the body from even the most malignant cerebral tumours are, however, rare. Some intrinsic tumours might be called 'relatively benign' in that they grow slowly and do not produce much destruction for many years. Some extrinsic tumours may become malignant. All metastases, whether intrinsic or extrinsic, are, of course, malignant, and malignant tumours of nearby structures may invade the skull and spine—e.g. from the nasopharynx, or the mediastinum.

Oddly enough, tumours of nerve cells and fibres are so rare as to be not worth mentioning. The neoplasms grow instead from the supporting tissue—the glia (**gliomas**); the meninges (**meningiomas**); the linings of the ventricles (**ependymomas**); the sheaths of the nerves (**neurofibromas**); or the **pituitary** gland.

Features which are common to all tumours will be described first, followed by those special to the different types.

CEREBRAL TUMOURS

General Features

Intracranial neoplasms produce symptoms in three main ways. (a) As the skull is a rigid box almost filled with brain, any new mass growing large enough fills up the remaining space and then causes the pressure inside the skull to rise. Hence the term **'space-occupying lesion'.** (b) Secondly, a tumour may compress the ventricles or the narrow parts of the C.S.F. pathways and so dam up the flow of the C.S.F. This still continues to be formed, however, again causing pressure to be built up. (c) Thirdly, the tumour presses upon, or destroys, some part of the brain itself. This direct effect produces symptoms and signs which become *gradually* worse and more extensive as the tumour grows, in complete contrast to the *sudden* onset of a vascular catastrophe. Tumours may occasionally erode a blood vessel and cause local haemorrhage or thrombosis with a sudden increase of symptoms.

Increased Intracranial Pressure

The symptoms and signs of raised intracranial pressure consist of **headaches,** especially after lying flat, increased by coughing or stooping; **vomiting,** usually at the height of the headache; **diplopia; blurring of vision** on movement of the head; **slowing** of the **pulse**; increasing **drowsiness** progressing eventually to coma; **dilation** of the **pupils** which fail to react to light. The vital sign on examination is **papilloedema**—swelling of the optic disc as seen through an ophthalmoscope. The optic disc is the rounded area where the fibres of the optic nerve leave the eyeball, and high pressure inside the skull can be transmitted by back-pressure through the sheath surrounding the optic nerve.

Direct Effects on the Brain

The common results of local damage to the brain are either irritative—i.e. fits; or destructive, causing loss of function (e.g. paralysis) of some part of the opposite side of the body. In addition there are special features according to the lobe affected. If the tumour lies in the frontal lobe there are also loss of memory and changes in personality; if in the temporal or occipital lobes, it can damage the optic radiations so that vision is lost in the half of each visual field opposite the lesion (homonymous hemianopia). Tumours growing in the dominant hemisphere (i.e. the left hemisphere in most people) cause progressively increasing speech disturbance (dysphasia).

The fits may take the form of convulsions affecting all parts of the body, or they may be **focal fits** affecting, say, one forearm only. The nearer the surface the tumour lies, the more likely is it to produce such focal fits, but as it grows, the amount of the limb affected becomes greater, and it is common to find that after the twitching has ceased, that part of the body remains paralysed for some time. This is called **Todd's paralysis.** Fits need not consist of convulsions, however. Temporal lobe tumours cause sudden hallucinations of smell, taste, or vision. The patient may see a clear picture, or smell some vague aroma just before losing consciousness. He often says that he has a strong feeling that all this has happened before—the so-called déjà vu sensation. Fits arising in the sensory cortex of the parietal lobe may consist simply of sudden short-lived attacks of loss of sensation of one limb, or one side of the body, while those arising in the occipital lobe may consist merely of blobs or flashes of light. These must not be confused with migraine (see p. 129).

Tumours arising in the brain stem are more common in children than in adults; they cause progressively increasing paralysis of eye movements and of other cranial nerves, with loss of sensation of the face, and later difficulty in swallowing. Intrinsic brain stem tumours are invariably fatal, but have a long and sometimes relapsing course. The stem may be compressed by benign tumours growing nearby, which may be removed completely.

Tumours in the cerebellum cause unsteadiness (ataxia) of limbs on the same side as the tumour, and, because they block off the IVth ventricle, they produce signs of raised intracranial pressure very early. Tumours in the vermis of the cerebellum (p. 18) can cause severe ataxia when walking, but this disappears when the patient is examined when lying down so that some patients are suspected of 'putting it on'.

The Different Types of Cerebral Tumour (See Fig. 8.1)

Meningiomas. These are benign extrinsic tumours, growing from the arachnoid mater, irritating and compressing the surface of the brain. The patients usually have a long history of headaches, focal fits, and focal paralysis, but as they grow they produce all the general signs of a space-occupying lesion. They can, however, be completely removed, and the patient completely cured.

The Gliomas. Most cerebral tumours, unfortunately, fall into this group. Gliomas develop from the glial cells—the supporting tissue—which include **astrocytes, oligodendrocytes** and **microglia.** They are always intrinsic and produce signs partly by eating their way through the nerve cells and fibres, and partly by compressing surrounding tissue which they have not yet destroyed. They produce all and any of the general features of a cerebral tumour, but generally do so more rapidly than do meningiomas. **Astrocytomas** are, however, of varying malignancy, some being relatively benign tumours growing slowly over many years. Others grow exceedingly rapidly, taking only a few weeks or months. These highly malignant tumours are called **glioblastomas.** Cysts form in some astrocytomas, drainage of which may improve the patient considerably. One special type of cystic astrocytoma grows in the cerebellum, and, if treated, carries a very good prognosis.

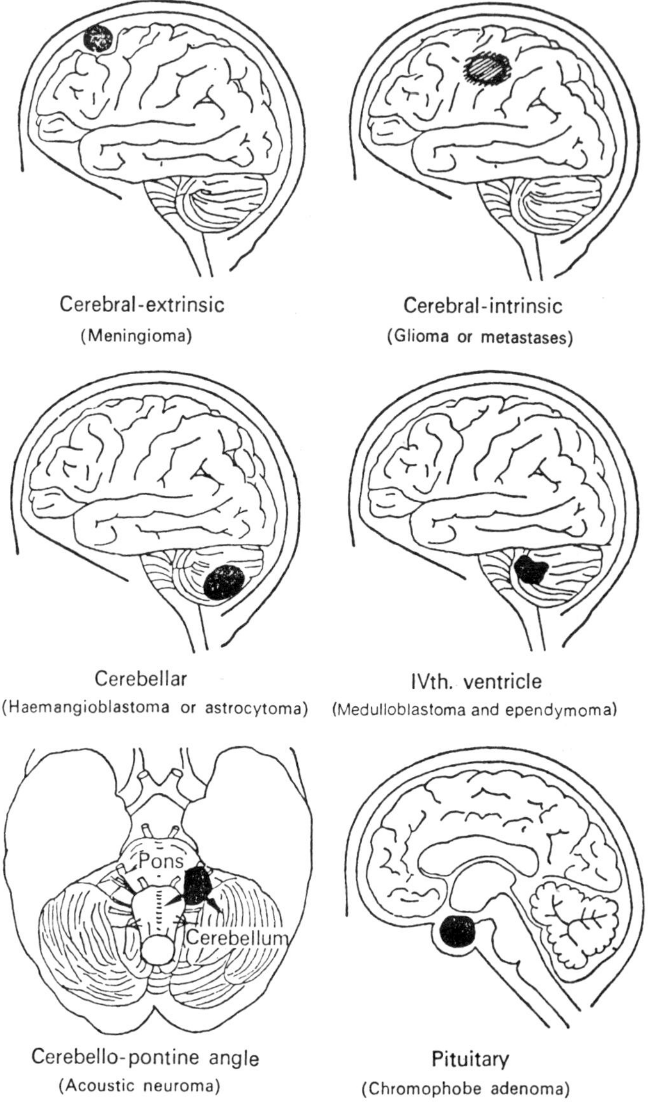

FIG. 8.1 The more common intracranial tumours and the positions in which they frequently occur. Metastases may occur anywhere.

The **oligodendrocytoma** is a very slow-growing tumour. It often has calcium laid down in it and this can be seen on a straight X-ray of the skull. Microgliomas are very rare.

The gliomas spread in amongst brain tissue and surgical removal means removing normal brain as well. Unless they lie in the extreme tip of the frontal, temporal, or occipital lobes, the patient is usually left with considerable disability, and the tumour is practically never completely removed. Sooner or later it grows again, but in the case of the slowly growing tumours, years of useful life may be given, so that these tumours are frequently operated upon.

Haemangioblastomas. This is a tumour of immature blood vessels; it almost invariably forms in the cerebellum, producing signs of raised intracranial pressure and marked ataxia. It tends to form a cyst, the tumour itself remaining as a little nodule in the cyst wall. Removal of cyst and nodule usually results in a complete cure.

Medulloblastomas. Almost confined to children under 12, this tumour develops from primitive cells in the roof of the **IVth ventricle** and spreads into the **cerebellum** and **brain stem.** It quickly blocks the C.S.F. pathways and causes all the signs of high intracranial pressure, and the children become increasingly ataxic. Surgical removal followed by deep X-ray therapy can give years of survival, but most cases eventually recur. These tumours are so near the C.S.F. pathways that they may throw off 'seedlings' which are carried down the spinal cord. X-ray treatment is often given to the spine as well, as a precaution against this. An **ependymoma** is another tumour which arises in the same area and behaves in the same way, but usually in rather older children. The results of excision are often better.

Acoustic Neuromas. Tumours grow from the sheath of the **VIIIth cranial nerve** and lie in the angle between the cerebellum and the pons (**cerebello-pontine angle**). They are benign, but because of their position, they compress the VIIIth nerve (producing deafness on that side), the VIIth nerve (producing some weakness of the face), and part of the Vth nerve (producing loss of sensation over the forehead and eye). They compress the cerebellum producing ataxia, and soon compress the brain stem, causing high intracranial pressure, and later causing bulbar paralysis and death. If diagnosed early enough they can be completely removed, though the operation usually leaves a facial paralysis, and of course, deafness on that side. Other tumours sometimes occur in a similar situation, including neurofibromas of the Vth nerve and meningiomas.

Pituitary Tumours. These form a rather special group. The pituitary gland lies in the **sella turcica** and is attached to the brain by the pituitary stalk. It contains three types of cells—**basophil**

cells, which stain blue; **eosinophil cells,** which stain red; and **chromophobe cells,** which 'fear colour' and do not stain. Each type of cell can produce a tumour. Minute tumours of the basophil cells form, but these are probably the result of a disturbance of the close relationship which exists between the pituitary and the adrenal glands, and they are found in association with tumours or hypertrophy of the adrenals. They cause the syndrome called **Cushing's syndrome.** This consists of **obesity, hairiness** of the face, stretching of the skin to produce **striae, amenorrhoea, hypertension** and **glycosuria.** Basophil adenomas are not space-occupying and treatment is usually directed at the adrenals.

Eosinophil adenomas cause increased output of growth hormones. If they develop before adult life, they produce **giants,** who nevertheless are physically rather feeble. If bone growth has stopped, they cause **acromegaly.** Acromegalics are easy to recognise. Their face, nose and jaw become large, wide spaces appear between the teeth, the skin coarsens and folds, and the hands and feet become progressively larger. These tumours can increase in size until they burst out of the sella and press on the optic chiasma, which lies just above, causing a **bitemporal hemianopia** (loss of the outer halves of both fields of vision). They can be removed, treated by implantation of radioactive material, or by deep X-ray.

Chromophobe adenomas are quite common, and grow to considerable size. Their cells have no special function, but because of their size they compress the rest of the pituitary, causing loss of hormones which this gland normally produces, and the state called **hypopituitarism.** The patients become feeble, with pale, round, yellowish, plump faces; they lose their body hair, feel the cold excessively, lose sexual desire and capacity, and women develop amenorrhoea. The tumours expand upwards and compress the chiasma, producing first a bitemporal hemianopia. If not treated, this will progress to blindness. The tumours can be removed surgically, treated by deep X-ray, or by implantation of radioactive substances. Irradiation in this area has, however, special dangers.

Metastatic Tumours. These can, of course, be deposited anywhere inside or outside the brain, and therefore are capable of producing any combination of signs and symptoms. They usually develop very rapidly, are almost always multiple, and practically never treatable. They most commonly arise from carcinoma of bronchus or breast, but they may give symptoms before the primary lesion is suspected or discovered.

The Diagnosis of Cerebral Tumours

The C.S.F. pressure is usually high, and though this can be shown by lumbar puncture, this is a *highly dangerous* procedure if a tumour is present, and the modern methods of diagnosis make it quite an unnecessary risk to take. **Brain scanning** (see p. 175) or the use of the **gamma-camera** after intravenous injection of a radioisotope, or in those centres possessing one, the **E.M.I. scanner** (see p. 176) will show the presence and location of most tumours affecting the cerebral hemispheres and by following this up with **carotid arteriography** (p. 174) the extent and often the exact nature of the tumour can be determined. In the brain stem, cerebellum or cerebello-pontine angle the various types of brain scanning and vertebral arteriography in very skilled hands can give similar information. **Ventriculography** (p. 174) is still commonly used though no longer as the primary examination. After locating its exact position, operative exploration will be required in most cases, to make certain of the type of tumour and to see whether removal is possible.

SPINAL TUMOURS

This term is used in neurology to mean tumours affecting the spinal cord, not tumours of the bones of the spine, though these may also sometimes grow to compress the cord itself.

Whereas most brain tumours are malignant, most spinal tumours are benign. There are five main types. **Neurofibromas** grow on the nerve roots; **meningiomas** grow from the arachnoid, and **haemangioblastomas** from immature blood vessels. All are benign and extrinsic, they compress the cord, but can be removed with complete cure. **Astrocytomas** and **ependymomas** grow in the substance of the cord. They are intrinsic and cannot be fully removed, but their rate of growth is very slow. Secondary deposits grow in the spaces around the cord, develop very rapidly, and attempts at removal or radiotherapy are rarely successful.

All spinal tumours produce similar symptoms, which depend on the level in the spine at which they develop. They are suspected when slowly progressive **paralysis** of the lower part of the body develops with a **clearcut level** on the skin below which sensation is lost. A neurofibroma may cause pain in the distribution of the nerve root for many months before it is big enough to compress the cord. At first it then causes a **Brown-Séquard syndrome** (see p. 40), and later, as it grows bigger, a **total transverse lesion.** Meningiomas and haemangioblastomas behave similarly, but with more cord signs, and less preliminary root pain.

The intrinsic tumours are most common in the cervical region. They first damage those sensory fibres which are crossing each other in the centre of the cord, and so produce a large patch of loss of sensation to pain and temperature over the arms and upper part of the body, very similar to syringomyelia (p. 98). Later they spread to involve the motor fibres in the pyramidal tracts and so cause paralysis of the lower limbs.

Tumours quite often develop below the cord itself in amongst the nerves forming the cauda equina. Because of their position, they cause a progressive flaccid paralysis of the legs with loss of sensation over the buttocks and backs of the legs, and paralysis of bladder and rectum. Nevertheless, if the tumour is benign and is not left too long before removal, all these signs are capable of recovery.

The diagnosis of spinal cord compression is confirmed by finding a block on the **Queckenstedt test** (see p. 171) on lumbar puncture, and usually a **high protein** in the C.S.F. Surgical exploration will be necessary, and in order to determine the exact position of the tumour, a **myelogram** (p. 176) will first be carried out. This must be done, for, on bedside examination alone, it is possible for a curable extrinsic tumour to masquerade as an inoperable intrinsic tumour, and the **exact** level of the tumour may not be possible to define by clinical examination alone.

PERIPHERAL NERVE TUMOURS

These rarely cause much trouble and consist almost entirely of neurofibromas. They may cause pain and sensory loss in the skin area that that nerve is going to supply, but usually they are symptomless. They can often be removed without sacrificing the nerve, but it is rarely necessary.

Von Recklinghausen's Disease

Large numbers of neurofibromas may occur throughout the body involving cranial, spinal and peripheral nerves. In such cases the skin is dark in colour, there are brown, so-called **'café-au-lait'** patches, and bluish naevi, together with numerous little wart-like tags called **mollusca fibrosa.** Sometimes these skin features are present alone, and the condition is often familial.

CONGENITAL TUMOURS

Congenital tumours may occur anywhere in the nervous system. They consist of **epidermoids, dermoids,** or **teratomas.** Epidermoids contain cheesy-like keratin. Dermoids may contain hair or teeth. Teratomas may have any type of human tissue. They all grow very slowly, and if conveniently situated may be completely removed.

Other space-occupying lesions due to aberrations in development include **chordomas,** which grow at the base of the skull causing considerable erosion of bone and compressing the brain stem and cranial nerves, and the **colloid cyst** which grows inside the IIIrd ventricle. Because of its position this soon causes blockage of the C.S.F. flow and symptoms of high pressure build up, at first intermittently on change of position, and then constantly. There are often mental changes, and curious episodes in which the legs suddenly give way (**drop attacks**). These tumours are all very rare.

Above the sella turcica and therefore close to the optic chiasma and the IIIrd ventricle, a **congenital cyst** called a **craniopharyngioma** can develop and cause signs of pressure on the local structures (e.g. the optic pathways). This is found sometimes in childhood, often not until adolescence or adult life. These cysts may **calcify** and be easily seen on straight X-rays.

Types of Intracranial and Spinal Tumour

Name	*Arising from*	*Benign or Malignant*
Meningioma	Arachnoid mater	Benign
Gliomas		
Astrocytoma	Astrocytes	Varies from low grade to high grade malignacy
Glioblastoma	Immature glial cells	The most malignant
Oligodendrocytoma	Oligodendrocytes	Low grade malignancy
Ependymoma	Ependymal cells lining ventricles	Low grade malignancy
Haemangioblastoma	Immature blood vessels	Benign
Medulloblastoma	Primitive cerebellar cells	Malignant
Neurofibroma or neurilemmoma	Sheaths of cranial or spinal nerves	Benign
Pituitary tumours	Pituitary cells	Usually benign
Eosinophil adenoma	Eosinophil cells	
Basophil adenoma	Basophil cells	
Chromophobe adenoma	Chromophobe cells	
Congenital Tumours		
Dermoids	Developing skin and subcutaneous tissue	Benign
Epidermoids	Developing epidermis	
Chordoma	Developing notochord	
Craniopharyngioma	Primitive nasopharynx	
Metastatic tumours (secondaries)	Usually from lung, breast, or alimentary tract	Malignant

Cysts may form in the arachnoid in the area of the temporal lobe and in the posterior fossa. These act as space-occupying lesions, yet when explored collapse so completely during the first stages of the operation that apparently nothing abnormal is found, and yet the patient is cured.

It must be realised that the term 'benign' refers to the behaviour of the tumour itself. The position in which it grows can at times cause as serious effects upon the patient as if it were malignant, but these are the tumours which offer real hope of complete removal.

9 *NEUROLOGICAL DISTURBANCES ASSOCIATED WITH SKELETAL ABNORMALITIES*

As brain and spinal cord are encased by the skull and the spine, and so many peripheral nerves run very close to bones, joints and ligaments, it is not surprising that skeletal abnormalities may sometimes involve nerve tissue. There are far too many possibilities to deal with individually, but there are certain conditions, commonly recurring, which are seen in every neurological and orthopaedic department.

INTERVERTEBRAL DISC DISEASE

The **discs** are 'cushions' of cartilage separating the vertebral bodies and held in place by a fibrous ring, the **annulus fibrosus,** which joins the bodies of the vertebrae together.

Acute Disc Prolapse

If the annulus ruptures, the disc will bulge through the gap, i.e. it will prolapse. In the cervical region this may compress the cord, causing an **acute quadriplegia.** This however is not common, and it is more likely to protrude slightly to one side, compressing a **nerve root** and causing severe pain down the arm. If a **thoracic disc** prolapses, there is so little room that it must compress the cord and cause a **paraplegia,** but fortunately this is rare. Prolapsed **lumbar discs** are, however, common. They miss the lower end of the cord and press on the lumbar and sacral nerves, causing **sciatica.** This consists of pain in the back, passing down the back of the thigh and either over the front of the lower leg towards the big toe (in L 4/5 lesions), or down the calf to the little toe (in L 5/S 1 lesions). Muscle spasm makes the back rigid, **scoliosis** develops, and straight-leg raising (**Lasègue's sign**) is limited on the affected side. Acute cervical and thoracic disc lesions require urgent operation, but 95% of lumbar disc lesions settle down on complete bed rest for 4-5 weeks. If severe symptoms persist, about 5% may require removal, when it is vitally important that the right level is operated upon. Occasionally a massive prolapse compresses the whole **cauda equina,** causing a **flaccid paraplegia** with urinary retention. Indeed signs of bladder disturbance in a patient with lumbago or sciatica is a warning of great importance. These patients require urgent operation.

Cervical Spondylosis

For many years it has been known that X-rays of the necks of people in middle age and older have shown degenerative changes in the discs with overgrowth of bone (**osteophytes**) forming hard bars. These were so common that doctors were reluctant to consider them responsible for any symptoms. More recently however it has been recognised that by compressing nerve roots, these spondylitic changes are responsible for most cases of 'fibrositis', 'rheumatism' or 'neuritis' in the shoulders and arms. The larger bars may press on the blood vessels supplying the anterior horn cells and pyramidal tracts in the cord and cause wasting and numbness in the arms with **progressive spastic paraparesis.** This type of case was once thought to be disseminated sclerosis of late onset.

Treatment is by **immobilisation** of the neck in a well-fitting collar for many months. **Neck manipulation is highly dangerous.** Only a few are suitable for surgery, which usually consists of a simple **decompression** to allow the cord to ride free of the bony spurs, but some surgeons are approaching the vertebral bodies from in front to try and avoid interference with the cord itself. Immobilisation may be made surgically permanent by fixing the spine with a **bone graft.**

THE CARPAL TUNNEL SYNDROME

As the **median nerve** enters the wrist to supply some of the muscles of the thumb and to give sensation to the thumb and first two fingers it passes through what is known as the **carpal tunnel.** In this, soft tissue and fat may become swollen and thickened resulting in compression of the nerve.

Carpal tunnel compression is particularly common in middle-aged women, causing them intolerable **pain, burning,** and **tingling** in the hand, especially during the **night,** waking them up, and leaving the thumb and first two fingers numb and weak while dressing in the morning. After a long time the muscles may waste. **Splinting** the wrist during the night gives relief to many people, and in others injections of **A.C.T.H.** or local infiltration of **hydrocortisone** may help; but the most certain means of cure is for the tunnel to be opened up surgically and the pressure relieved, the whole procedure being quite a minor operation.

Occasionally other nerves, such as the ulnar, or the nerves to the feet, are similarly trapped, when the general term **entrapment neuropathy** is used. These others are rare, but the treatment is the same. The exact site of an entrapment can be determined by nerve conduction studies using the electromyograph (see p. 178) so that unnecessary operations can be avoided.

THE THORACIC OUTLET SYNDROME

Many cases previously given this name were either due to cervical disc or carpal tunnel compression, but in some patients, as the nerves pass through the **root of the neck** to reach the arms, they are compressed by **tight bands** of **muscle** in this area. These patients, again mainly women, after carrying heavy weights, or after increase in body weight with drooping of the shoulders, develop painful tinglings throughout the whole arm. Some are helped by physiotherapy to correct their posture; others need division of the muscle bands, but the diagnosis is now made less frequently, and the procedure is less common. A similar situation arises if the angle between the clavicle and the first rib is abnormally narrow (the costo-clavicular syndrome).

CERVICAL RIBS

It is convenient to consider these congenital anomalies here. They are **small ribs** attached to the 7th cervical vertebrae, and because of their position they **raise** and **stretch** the nerves which normally run over the first rib. This results in wasting of the small muscles of the hand, and loss of sensation over the little and ring fingers and part of the forearm. If the symptoms are severe enough, these small ribs can be removed.

PRESSURE NEUROPATHIES

Certain nerves, especially the **ulnar** at the **elbow** and the **external popliteal** outside the **knee,** are superficial, and may be compressed simply by resting on them for long periods of time, especially in thin people, those whose blood vessels show degenerative changes (e.g. in old age), in diabetic patients, and when nearby joints have been deformed by an old injury. This may occur during a long period in bed, or by the application of an inadequately padded plaster cast, or by the use of adhesive materials over the lower legs for skin traction. The hand will waste and sensation be lost over the ring and little finger, or if in the leg, there will be a **foot drop.** Though most of these recover, they should never have been allowed to occur, and prevention of this by adequate protection of the nerves is the responsibility of the doctor and nurse.

BONY ABNORMALITIES

At the Base of the Skull

The skull base and posterior fossa may be unusually flat. This is called **platybasia,** and need not be important, but it is often associated with **basilar invagination** or **basilar impression.** This is important, for it is as if the skull were pressed downwards on the cervical spine, the first cervical vertebra (the atlas) being almost inside the posterior fossa, which is in turn so shallow that parts of the cerebellum (**the cerebellar tonsils**) are squeezed down through the foramen magnum (cerebellar ectopia). These patients who have a short neck, and a low hair line, become **increasingly ataxic.** The bony abnormality may be congenital or the result of softening of bone as in **Paget's disease.** Basilar impression is also often associated with the **Arnold-Chiari deformity** and **syringomyelia,** both of which are described in Chapter 10.

Kypho-scoliosis

As the spinal cord runs in the spinal canal it is obvious that if the **canal** is **distorted** in any way the cord and its dural sheath will itself be distorted, and this may reach such a degree as to cause damage to the nerve fibres. This can occur in severe scoliosis producing a **progressive spastic weakness** of the legs. Great care in diagnosis is required however for some neurological lesions, such as **syringomyelia** (p. 98), may cause muscle imbalance and scoliosis and the neurological signs may be more the result of the primary disease than of the bony deformity.

10 *CONGENITAL MALFORMATIONS*

Why some children are born with developmental defects is usually a mystery. It is obvious that if the developing foetus is damaged there will be some sort of abnormality at birth, but what that abnormality is depends not only on the site of the damage, but on the stage of development at which it occurs. What causes the damage, however, is usually unknown. Various things have been suggested, all acting on the mother—virus infections (especially German measles), exposure to X-rays, injury, heredity, even psychological causes. In fact there is rarely a proven cause, though the drug Thalidomide was shown to cause deformities if given in the early stages of pregnancy, and a few other drugs are under suspicion.

Babies may be born with gross defects of the nervous system such as the absence of a brain (**anencephalic monster**) but they do not survive long. In others the head and brain may be abnormally small (**microcephaly**). The children are mentally defective and perhaps epileptic, but they survive normally. The defect that most frequently requires attention, however, is when the head appears abnormally large (**hydrocephalus**).

Hydrocephalus (Fig. 10.1)

The lay phrase 'water on the brain' is not a bad description, for this condition is due to the presence of too much C.S.F. at too high a pressure. This causes a baby's head to enlarge, for the bones are free to separate at the sutures. By adult life the sutures are closed and this cannot happen, so that symptoms of raised intracranial pressure would develop instead (see p. 79).

Hydrocephalus can be present at birth (congenital) or may develop from various causes later (acquired). There are two types, **obstructive** and **communicating.** If the C.S.F., after being formed in the lateral ventricles, cannot pass through the ventricular system owing to an obstruction in the IIIrd ventricle, aqueduct, or IVth ventricle, the lateral ventricles enlarge, and blow up the brain like a balloon, the cortex becoming stretched and at times almost paper-thin. This is called obstructive hydrocephalus (Fig. 10.1b), the pressure being highest in the ventricles and will occur for instance if the C.S.F. pathways are particularly narrow, as in stenosis of the aqueduct.

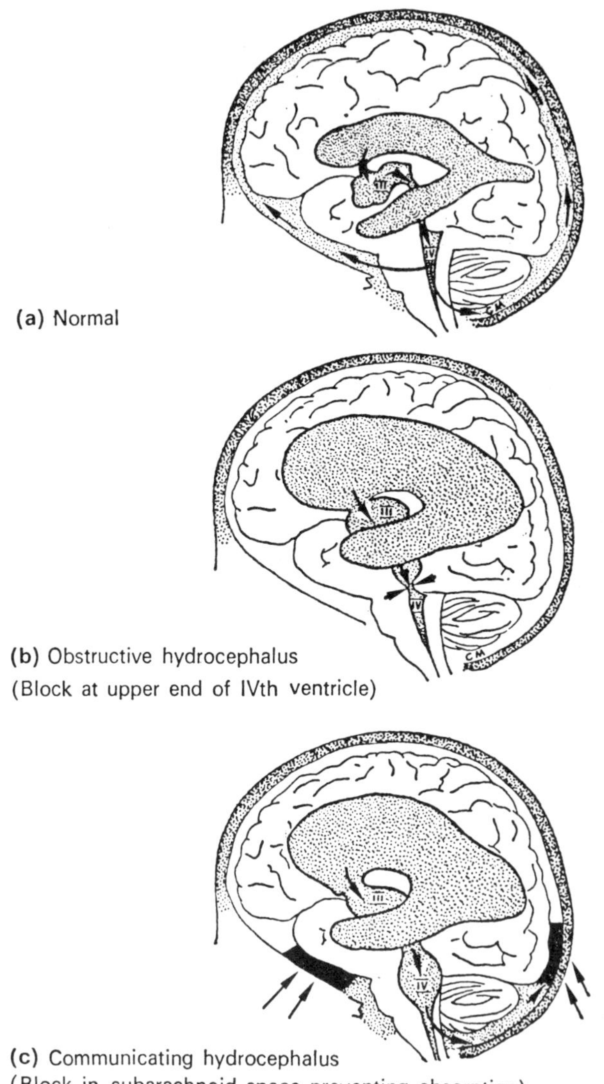

FIG. 10.1 Hydrocephalus. The ventricles are drawn as if it were possible to see through the brain substance.

If, however, the C.S.F. can get out of the ventricular system, but owing to blockage in the subarachnoid space cannot then circulate properly to reach the upper surface of the brain where it is absorbed, the pressure then builds up outside the brain as well. This is termed communicating hydrocephalus (Fig 10.1c) and can occur if there are **adhesions** or thickening in the subarachnoid spaces due to **past inflammation** (e.g. meningitis) or due to haemorrhage into the subarachnoid space—an event which can cause hydrocephalus in adults as well.

In either event the ventricles become enlarged and the terms internal and external hydrocephalus, sometimes used, are not entirely satisfactory.

Hydrocephalus may be present at birth (presenting mechanical difficulties), or it may develop later. The head is large, the fontanelles remain wide open, and even bulging, and by charting the circumference of the head progressive enlargement can be measured. The sutures can be felt to be separated, the forehead is bossed and the eyes may be pushed downwards, the whole head often being too heavy for the child to hold up. Mental retardation is frequent, but surprisingly high intelligence is sometimes possible, and in milder cases some sort of balance develops between the formation of C.S.F. and the defect in its absorption, and the pressure does not go on increasing. We then speak of an arrested hydrocephalus, and in these cases normal intelligence is possible. It is for this reason that attempts are always being made to treat the condition before irreparable damage has been done by stretching and thinning of the brain.

Investigation and Treatment

A method adopted for many years was to inject a dye into the lateral ventricle through the enlarged fontanelle and if a few minutes afterwards this can be shown to have reached the lumbar C.S.F. (by doing a lumbar puncture), the fluid must have been able to get out of the ventricular system and the hydrocephalus must be a communicating one. This was not particularly reliable, however, and did not show, for instance, if there were partial stenosis of the pathways but not complete obstruction. There is also a danger in doing a lumbar puncture in obstructive hydrocephalus as there is in high pressure due to intracranial tumours.

X-rays are now more frequently used. The introduction of air or an opaque fluid into the ventricle then allows photographs to be taken and by positioning of the head the **exact site** and sometimes the nature of the **block** can be demonstrated and examined on X-ray plates at leisure. C.A.T. scans may replace these techniques.

The aim of treatment is to **bypass** the **block** and lead the fluid from the lateral ventricles where it is formed to somewhere where it may be absorbed. An opening may be made in the wall of the IIIrd ventricle (**IIIrd ventriculostomy**). This is now very rarely carried out because the opening would close up again so easily. A tube may be led from the lateral ventricle through a burr-hole under the scalp and into the cisterna magna (**Torkildsen's procedure**). This is a good procedure but the tube often blocks and if the C.S.F. obstruction is in the subarachnoid space it cannot get out of the cisterna magna either. For this reason the **Spitz-Holter** and **Pudenz valves** have been developed and the use of these is described in details on pages 164–5.

These procedures are of value in hydrocephalus which is increasing. An arrested hydrocephalus is best left alone. The children may develop normally, or may do so in a retarded manner, but they are very prone to infection, and many used to succumb to tuberculous meningitis.

Craniosynostosis

In hydrocephalus the skull sutures are so widely separated that they cannot fuse, but in **craniosynostosis,** commonly called craniostenosis, the sutures **fuse** too **early,** the **fontanelles** are **closed** perhaps before the baby is born. Sometimes one suture is involved, sometimes several. If the sagittal suture is involved the skull develops a shape like an inverted 'V'—**turricephaly.** If both the coronal sutures are fused the skull cannot expand to contain the growing brain. Pressure builds up and is transmitted to the orbits producing marked **prominence of the eyes.** There are often **other congenital deformities** such as webbed fingers, cleft palate and bronchiectasis. Surgical treatment is required urgently in the first few weeks of life to prevent the complications of high pressure, the sutures are separated and attempts made to prevent them re-fusing by coating the edges with plastic or by inserting tantalum foil. The results are very variable, sometimes excellent, but sometimes whatever is done the sutures seem to re-fuse.

Spina Bifida Occulta

During development of the spine, the **neural arch,** i.e. the arch formed by the two laminae and the spinous process, may fail to join in the centre (Fig. 10.2). This condition is called **spina bifida,** and X-rays, especially of the lumbo-sacral region, may show a gap where the spinous process should be. If this is only detected by X-ray it is called spina bifida occulta (hidden); it may affect one or several spines, and is usually without significance. Very occasionally, however, there is also a defect in the development of the nervous tissue underneath. This may be accompanied by deformities of the feet (e.g. pes cavus) or difficulty in control of urine.

Some patients with a spina bifida have a **naevus** on the overlying skin, and perhaps tufts of hair growing on it. In many of these there is a track leading from this into the theca and ending in a **lipoma** or **dermoid.** They may compress the cord or the cauda equina, and act as a spinal tumour, or because there is a connection between the spinal theca and the skin infection may enter resulting in repeated attacks of meningitis. These tracks can be removed surgically.

Meningoceles

If the gap in the bony covering of the nervous system is large enough, a bulge of the meninges may project under the skin (Fig.

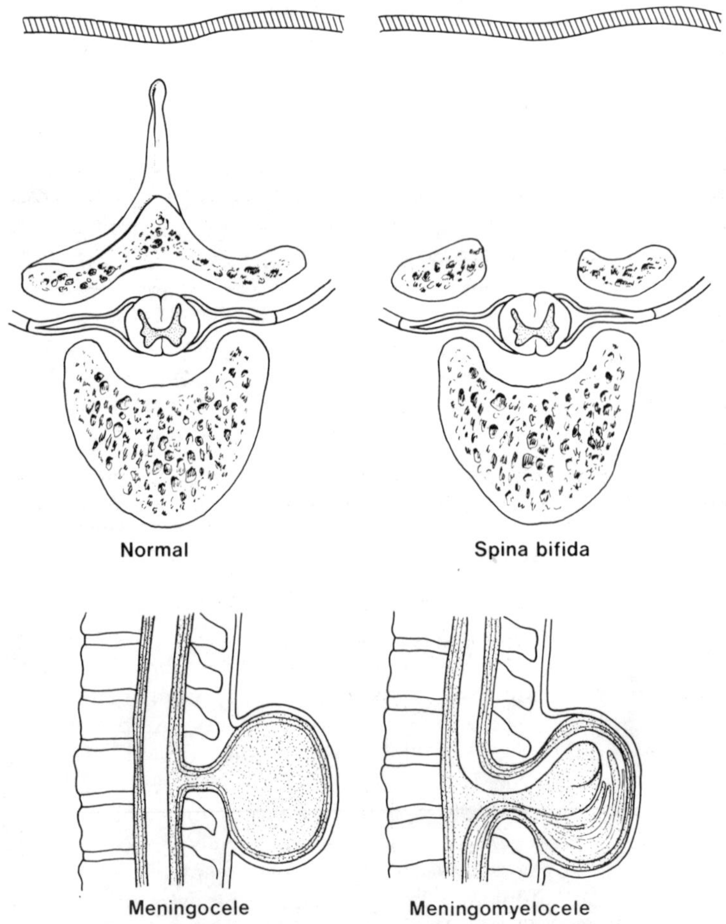

FIG. 10.2 Spina bifida, meningocele and meningomyelocele.

10.2). This may occur in any part of the spine, but is most common in the lumbar region or at, or just below, the occiput. Part of the spinal cord and spinal nerves may also enter such a sac, forming a meningomyelocele. These infants often have mal-developed, deformed and paralysed lower limbs. The temptation to excise these sacs and close the skin over the defect is very great, and indeed may have to be carried out to avoid rupture and meningeal infection. However, sometimes hydrocephalus develops after this procedure. Whether this is because a sort of escape valve has been removed, or whether they were becoming hydrocephalic anyway, is not always clear, for some of these children also have the Arnold-Chiari deformity, see below (Fig. 10.3). If the myelocele is excised there may, of course, be permanent paralysis of the legs, but some surgeons accept this, and then train the child at a paraplegic centre from an early age; others claim good results simply from closing the defect and correcting the deformities of the limbs.

Surgeons are faced with great problems in deciding whether to allow children with some of these congenital abnormalities to deteriorate rapidly, or whether to undertake a procedure which allows the infant to survive but leaves him mentally defective or paralysed. Religious, emotional, humanitarian and social aspects all arise and may point in different directions, so that hard and fast rules cannot be made. Each case has to be considered separately, and the parents guided by a wise and sympathetic surgeon.

Cerebellar Ectopia and the Arnold-Chiari Deformity (see Fig. 10.3)

Several **foramen magnum deformities** are included under these headings. To begin with there is often a bony deformity such as

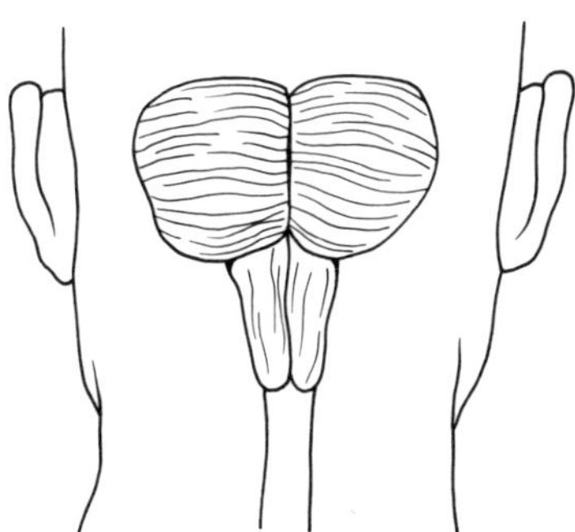

FIG. 10.3 Elongated tonsils in Arnold-Chiari deformity.

basilar invagination (see Chap. 9) or fusion of one or more cervical vertebrae (**Klippel Feil syndrome**). In the simplest form the cerebellar tonsils are prolapsed through the foramen magnum into the cervical region (**cerebellar ectopia**). There is, however, very little room so that they compress the cord and cause both **ataxia** and **weakness** in the arms and legs. In infants the circulation of the C.S.F. is also impeded so that there is a resultant **hydrocephalus.** Once thought to be a rarity, especially in adults, this is now diagnosed quite frequently in neurological practice, and it is important to recognise it because surgical **decompression** of the area may relieve a progressive disability.

This also applies to the complete **Arnold-Chiari deformity** where not only are the tonsils prolapsed, but the medulla is elongated into the cervical region, there is a mound pushing the medulla backwards and the nerve roots in the upper cervical region (which are normally horizontal) have to travel upwards to reach the foramina through which the spinal nerves emerge.

Perhaps the most important aspect of this and similar anomalies in this area is that it may be responsible for the formation of **cavities** in the centre of the spinal cord, i.e. for the condition known as **syringomyelia** which is described below.

SYRINGOMYELIA

The amount of argument that has waxed and waned over the last twenty years or so about the aetiology and classification of this condition has been such that no-one need be blamed for feeling somewhat confused.

Syringomyelia is a condition in which a **cavity** or **syrinx** forms in the centre of the cervical cord and/or the lower brain stem (**syringobulbia**) and may even extend as far as the lumbar region. For many years this was classified as a degenerative disease for which there was no useful treatment.

However, careful investigations by means of neuroradiology and exploration of the area by neurosurgeons have now shown that in the majority of cases there is an **anomaly** at the **foramen magnum,** the **tonsils** are **prolapsed** while the roof foramen (the **foramen of Magendie**) from which the C.S.F. should escape from the ventricle to enter the subarachnoid space, is **closed.** As a result the fluid is thrust down the central canal of the cord (see p. 19) expanding it and resulting in irregular cavitation around it. The lesion is so placed (see Fig. 10.4) that it damages the **pain** and **temperature fibres** as they cross from their point of entry to the opposite spinothalamic tract (see p. 25). Later the anterior horn cells and then the pyramidal tracts are involved.

Symptoms

The patients, usually aged 20-45, first notice either that their hands are becoming thinner, or that they are **burning** or cutting their fingers **without** noticing the heat or the **pain,** the appearance of a

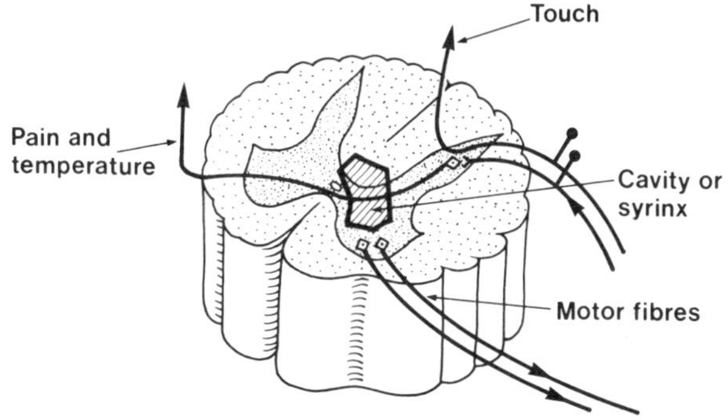

FIG. 10.4 The site of the lesion in syringomyelia. Note how, by lying in the centre of the cord, it can involve both the anterior horn cells and the crossing fibres of pain and temperature, while those for touch escape.

blister or septic sore being the first sign that anything has happened. The hands and arms become very **wasted,** cold and blue, and both wasting and **sensory loss** may extend to the rest of the body, including the tongue. In the later stages, the legs may become stiff as the pyramidal tracts are involved.

Signs

Wasting is usually present in the hand muscles, the forearms and shoulder girdles, and the hands show scars from **old burns** and cuts. There is loss of sensation to **pain** and **temperature** over the arms, shoulders, upper chest and often the occiput, but above and below these areas sensation may be normal. Characteristically, despite the degree of sensory loss, light touch can still be felt in the affected areas, producing what is known as **dissociated sensory loss.** The **reflexes** are **absent** in the arms, but later, if the cavity is large enough, it affects the pyramidal tracts and the legs will show increased tone, increased reflexes and **extensor plantars.**

Treatment

No drug therapy is available, and deep X-ray therapy, once popular, is more dangerous than useful. If careful myelography (see p. 176) shows the anomalies mentioned above to be present, then surgical decompression of the foramen magnum and upper cervical region, with or without incision of a large syrinx, may halt what is otherwise an inevitably progressive disease.

Some may be confused by hearing the terms **'communicating'** and **'non-communicating'** syringomyelia used. Syringomyelia as it has been described is the 'communicating' variety in that the cavity communicates with the ventricles. Cavities can, however, form in the cord as the result of trauma, of breakdown of tumours and several other acquired, not congenital, conditions. It is this cavity which is described by some as non-communicating syringomyelia, but it would be much wiser to limit the use of the word syringomyelia to the so-called 'communicating' type.

11 *THE DEMYELINATIVE DISEASES*

The Meaning of Demyelination

Myelin is a substance which forms the sheath covering the majority of nerve fibres, whether they lie within the brain and spinal cord, or run outside these structures in the cranial and spinal peripheral nerves. When myelin-sheathed (i.e. **myelinated**) fibres are collected together the tissue looks white, and it is this that forms the white matter of the brain and spinal cord.

Almost any damage to nervous tissue can cause these sheaths to degenerate, but there are certain diseases in which this seems to happen spontaneously without the exact cause being known. Loss of the myelin sheath is termed **demyelination.** Without its myelin the nerve fibre (or axon) does not conduct impulses properly so that there is loss of function in the part of the body supplied. The best known of the apparently spontaneously developing demyelinative diseases is **disseminated** (or **multiple**) **sclerosis.**

If only the myelin sheath is damaged, it can form again, so that after a period of time function will be restored to the nerve fibre. If, however, the disease process has destroyed the nerve fibre (or axon) as well, then recovery is less likely. Nerve fibres can, of course, grow again, as is seen following peripheral nerve injuries, but often **scar tissue** forms, preventing proper re-growth and recovery. Scar tissue is formed after injury in the central nervous system, too, in this case by the glial cells, the process being called **gliosis.** Though strictly speaking a healing process, all scar tissue gradually shrinks, and in doing so it may draw nearby healthy tissue into the area of gliosis. This causes slowly progressive disability without necessarily any new flare-up of the disease. It will be easier to understand what happens in the demyelinative diseases if these few facts are borne in mind.

Disseminated or Multiple Sclerosis

Sclerosis is 'hardening'. When post-mortems are carried out in this disease, hard areas of **gliosis** are found scattered or 'disseminated' throughout the central nervous system. The cause of the disease, however, remains unknown. Various factors have been suggested. Today it is believed by many that a **'slow virus'** acquired in early years and taking many years to produce symptoms may be responsible. This is far from certain. That this might be a form of measles virus is considered by some, but evidence to support this is quite absent in many cases. **Allergy,** or a **hypersensitivity** reaction to various different infective or toxic factors is a popular theory and in the minds of many the most likely, but others believe in influences coming from diet, climate, toxins, thrombosis of small veins and hereditary susceptibility. None seems to bear any consistent relationship, but familial incidence of the disease is not uncommon and there may well be some **inherited abnormality** of the way in which nerve tissue resists an infection.

It usually starts in **young adult** life, occasionally in adolescents or even young children, and very occasionally occurs for the first time in middle life. It rarely begins over the age of 50. Women are slightly more often affected than men, and country dwellers more than town dwellers. It is a disease of **temperate climates,** very rare in the Tropics, India, or the West Indies, and rare in Australia and South Africa except in first generation immigrants from countries frequently affected.

Patches of demyelination—so-called **'plaques'**—develop in some part of the spinal cord, cerebellum, brain stem, cerebral hemispheres, or optic pathways. The peripheral nerves are not affected. These patches flare up, then take weeks or months to settle down, and after an interval of months or years, flare up again in some other site. After several attacks the healing process of gliosis upsets all attempts at re-myelination, and permanent 'sclerosis' and loss of function results.

Symptoms

The course of the disease is characterised by a series of **relapses** and **remissions.** The symptoms of each relapse depend upon the sites where the plaques of demyelination occur. There may be blurring, or complete loss of **vision,** in one eye; paralysis of eye movement and **double vision; numbness, weakness** and **clumsiness** of one or both arms or legs; slurring of **speech; unsteadiness** of the hands or legs; or urgency and increased frequency of **micturition.** Any one of these symptoms may occur by itself, or together with any or all of the others. They may last several weeks, or even several months (never several hours), and then clear up, and the patient may be quite well for months or years and is said to have a 'remission'. There is then another episode (a relapse) which may involve the same, or some entirely different, part of the nervous system. Recovery this time, during the remission, may not be so complete, and following the next relapse, the patient may make only **partial recovery** and so on.

However, the gloomy picture which is normally painted of progressive disability to a bed-ridden state is not necessarily always true. The disease may consist of mild relapses and long remissions throughout life, with very little permanent effects. Others have a series of relapses, with some residual disability, and then further deterioration ceases. There are, of course, cases in which each relapse worsens the condition until the patient becomes bed-ridden and incontinent in early middle life; and a further group of cases who are so severely affected from the very beginning that they progress very rapidly and become grossly disabled within a year—but even they may then remain in this state for many years. It is not in itself a killing disease and the prognosis in many cases is much better than is usually believed. This has given rise to the recognition of a **'benign relapsing variety'** of the disease—the existence of which should be stressed to any young patient facing the future with alarm.

Signs

When a patient is examined many more abnormal signs are often found than the symptoms might suggest. The optic disc seen through the ophthalmoscope may be abnormally pale, even without a history of visual disturbance; one or other of the eye muscles may be weak, causing diplopia; the eyes often show that rhythmical oscillation seen in cerebellar and brain stem disease, called **nystagmus**; the speech is slurred (**dysarthria**); the limbs show a mixture of cerebellar signs, producing **ataxia,** and upper motor neurone signs, producing weakness, **spasticity,** exaggerated reflexes and extensor plantars. In addition, there is an odd mental attitude termed **euphoria,** in which the patient appears cheerfully unconcerned about what is often gross disability. There are very few diseases which involve so many parts of the central nervous system, and it is this finding in a young patient that raises the suspicion of disseminated sclerosis in a doctor's mind.

Treatment

No curative treatment has yet been found, and because relapses tend to clear up by themselves, it is very difficult to know if any drug being given at that time has been beneficial. There is little doubt however that in the acute stages of a relapse a course of **A.C.T.H.** injections will often produce a more rapid and more marked improvement than would have been expected naturally. Unfortunately the long-term use of A.C.T.H. or cortisone does not prevent further relapses. Spasticity and flexor spasms can be reduced by the use of diazepam and by the drug lioresal, but this is merely treating a symptom. Many other drugs have been used, including arsenic, copper, Vitamin B.12, vaccines from Russia and elsewhere, and countless unconventional remedies, but any apparent beneficial effect they may have is due either to a **spontaneous remission,** or the feeling that something is being done, or both.

In recent years various diets have been given publicity, e.g. gluten free, sunflower seed etc. but most neurologists consider that there is no real evidence of benefit and certainly none for the advanced case who longs for *some* help.

As a result of this, patients tend to go from specialist to specialist, seeking new advice and new treatment, and are very liable to fall into unscrupulous hands. There are, however, mixed medical and lay organisations, such as the **Multiple Sclerosis Society,** which have branches in all larger cities and towns, and which, if well guided, can do much to aid the social problems of these patients. The British Red Cross and the local authorities produce many aids to nursing, mobility, personal hygiene and household management, which greatly ease the burden of disability, and enable the patient to fill a useful role in the community.

Retro-bulbar Neuritis (Optic Neuritis)

This condition is usually due to a patch of **demyelination** developing in one **optic nerve,** and is most commonly an early stage of disseminated sclerosis. Later on the other nerve may be affected, and occasionally both at once.

Symptoms

The patient first develops **pain** in one eye, and it hurts to move it or to press on it. The **vision** then very quickly becomes blurred, particularly in its **central** part, and this may progress to total loss of vision. However, after a few days it begins to recover and within a matter of weeks or months the vision may be completely normal. In some cases, however, a little area of permanently impaired vision remains in the centre of the field, which interferes greatly with reading, writing, sewing, etc.

Signs

If the patch develops in the nerve just behind the globe (i.e. **retro-bulbar**), mild swelling of the optic disc can be seen through the ophthalmoscope. This is sometimes called **papillitis.** After the acute stage some nerve fibres atrophy and the disc then looks pale, or even dead white (**optic atrophy**). If the patch develops further back along the nerve, there may be no swelling, but the atrophy can still develop later. By charting the visual fields the blind area can be demonstrated in the centre—the so-called **central scotoma.**

Treatment

A.C.T.H. and cortisone often hasten the improvement, and are worth using, for the sooner the acute stage settles down, the less chance there is of permanent visual impairment.

Transverse Myelitis

During one of the relapses of disseminated sclerosis, a plaque of demyelination may extend across the spinal cord, producing a **transverse cord lesion** (see p. 40). Sometimes, however, this will occur without any other evidence of disseminated sclerosis. The lesion is usually in the thoracic region, and the cause is unknown.

Symptoms

After a preliminary period of pain around the lower thoracic or abdominal regions (which may be mistaken for pleurisy, cholecystitis, or appendicitis), there is rapid weakness and loss of sensation in the legs, with retention of urine.

Signs

At the very beginning, especially in children, there may be a flaccid paralysis of the legs, but soon this becomes spastic with exaggerated reflexes and extensor plantars. All forms of sensation are lost below a clear cut level on the trunk. Bed sores and urinary infection are very likely to occur.

Treatment

Though A.C.T.H. may help in the acute stage, the treatment is usually that of careful nursing of a paraplegic patient. The prognosis varies in different cases. There may be complete recovery, or gross residual spastic paraplegia. The sooner movement begins to return the better the outlook, for total paralysis for over a month carries a very serious prognosis.

Bilateral Retro-bulbar Neuritis and Transverse Myelitis

There is a rare condition called **neuro-myelitis optica,** or Devic's disease, where the patient develops retro-bulbar neuritis in both eyes, not necessarily together, followed soon by a transverse myelitis. It is probably a variety of disseminated sclerosis, but if recovery takes place from the acute stage, there is not the same tendency for relapses to occur.

Demyelinative Lesions in Infants

Large areas of **demyelination** can occur in the cerebral hemispheres in infants, particularly in the **occipital** lobes. They result in the acute onset of **fits,** rapidly developing **blindness,** and often spastic paralysis, the whole picture progressing slowly to total disability. The condition is called **Schilder's disease.** There are several varieties in which the differences are rather slight clinically and mainly of interest to the pathologist.

A.C.T.H. given in the acute stage may help to prevent gross disability, but many cases have had too extensive a lesion for useful improvement to take place.

The Cerebro-spinal Fluid in Demyelinative Disease

In the chronic stages of these diseases the C.S.F. may be quite normal. In the acute stages there is often a rise in the lymphocyte count, usually less than 100 per cu mm, and a slight rise in protein. The Lange curve may show a paretic pattern (see p. 193), but the W.R. is always negative. It is now known that in disseminated sclerosis, even when the cells and protein are normal, if the types of protein are separated out by the process called electrophoresis, the gamma-globulin portion may rise from less than 10% of the total protein to 15–30% and if facilities are available a marked rise may be shown in what is called the IgG fraction. These estimations can be very valuable in diagnosis.

The Influence of Pregnancy on Demyelinative Disease

Patients with disseminated sclerosis are usually very well during pregnancy, but there is often a relapse during the puerperium. This however may be followed by a very prolonged remission so that there is not a great deal of evidence that pregnancy makes things much worse in the long run. It is of course clear that the responsibility of a large family should not be in the hands of a mother who is becoming progressively handicapped, but it is not justified to advise a young woman never to have a child, and the danger of passing the disease on is so slight that this should not be a reason for avoiding marriage or childbirth. It has not yet been clearly defined if the oral contraceptives have any influence on the course of disseminated sclerosis.

12 DEGENERATIVE DISEASES

Cells and fibres sometimes cease to function, shrink and gradually disappear, for no known reason. This process is rather vaguely called **degeneration.** Changes of this sort can undoubtedly occur in the nervous system as a result of ischaemia from narrowing of blood vessels in arteriosclerosis, but often all other systems are normal, and yet certain parts of the brain or spinal cord die. The degenerative process may be diffuse, or it may pick out particular parts of the nervous system, and so result in symptoms and signs which when collected together form syndromes, which can easily be recognised. These include **Parkinsonism, motor-neurone disease,** and the **cerebral atrophies.**

Parkinsonism

James Parkinson was a general practitioner who first described the 'shaking palsy', which later came to be known as **paralysis agitans.** Its features are due to degeneration of nerve cells in the **extra-pyramidal system**—the basal ganglia and nuclei in the upper brain stem. There are several varieties of the disease; (a) **paralysis agitans** itself, the cause of which is unknown; (b) **post-encephalitic Parkinsonism,** following some years after an encephalitis, particularly encephalitis lethargica; (c) **arteriosclerotic Parkinsonism,** due to defective blood supply to the basal nuclei; (d) patients receiving very high dosage of certain **tranquilliser** drugs—therefore often to be seen in mental institutions; (e) **post-traumatic Parkinsonism** when the same parts of the brain have been directly injured or rendered short of oxygen in prolonged coma (a similar state follows carbon monoxide—coal gas—poisoning); and (f) **syphilitic Parkinsonism**—a rare complication of syphilis, now hardly ever seen.

Symptoms

The three main symptoms are **tremor, rigidity** of the muscles, and **akinesia,** i.e. the inability to initiate movements or to perform them quickly enough. Any one of these may predominate. *Paralysis agitans* begins in middle life, with first a **slowing up** of all movements, together with aching in the shoulders and arms; as rigidity and akinesia increase it becomes difficult to raise the arms (e.g. for doing the back of the hair), to get out of a chair, or to turn suddenly. The writing becomes progressively smaller, the **speech monotonous** and indistinct.

In other cases, the first symptom is the tremor. This may start in the thumb and hand on one side, and then gradually progress to involve the wrist, the other arm and later the legs. The tremor is worst when the patient is trying to remain still, but over the years it gradually increases until it becomes so marked that it is impossible to control it or conceal it.

In most cases both tremor, rigidity and akinesia develop together.

The autonomic system is also disturbed as shown by excessive formation of **saliva, sweating** and greasiness of the skin. There is intractable **constipation.** In the late stages, the memory deteriorates and obsessional trends develop, which often refer mainly to the bowel habits. To their relatives the patients become irritable, querulous and never satisfied, though superficially to the outsider they appear to remain remarkably cheerful in face of distressing disability.

Signs

A fully developed case is unmistakeable. The face shows no changes of expression, and blinking is infrequent. This **'mask-like'** appearance can usually be transformed by a smile. Owing to the muscular rigidity the patient walks with **small shuffling steps,** stooped forwards, arms and legs bent, and the arms held across the body instead of swinging in the normal manner. The rapid movements needed to correct a sudden change of position are impossible, so that, if the patient is given a slight push, he will appear to trot forwards more and more quickly. This is called **'propulsion'.** The rigidity can be felt by moving a joint, when it gives a jerky sensation like a **cog-wheel.**

The **tremor** is most obvious in the fingers, hands and wrist, but may affect any part of the body, including the head, chin and tongue. It is **rhythmical** and **regular,** but stops as soon as the limb is put into action, and starts again when at rest. **Speaking** produces rapid, **monotonous** runs of words, at times almost indistinguishable. Despite all this, the mind may remain quite clear and there are many who, having had the disease for many years, are able to manage large and profitable businesses.

Post-encephalitic Parkinsonism affects **younger** people, is often mainly unilateral, and is more likely to produce mental change. These patients may have striking attacks called **oculogyric crises.** In these the eyes (and sometimes the head) appear to be forced to turn upwards for minutes at a time, without any loss of consciousness. There is a history of **encephalitis,** or of a serious illness which could have been an encephalitis. Oculogyric crises may follow an overdose of certain tranquillisers.

Arteriosclerotic Parkinsonism affects the **later** age groups. The onset is often abrupt and rigidity is less.

Syphilitic Parkinsonism can only be diagnosed if there is a clear history of syphilis or the patient has a **positive W.R.**

Treatment

Belladonna used to be the main drug, but now there are a number of more effective remedies. These include anti-spasmodics such as **benzhexol (Artane), orphenadrine (Disipal),** and many other drugs with a confusing complexity of names, the number showing that none was truly satisfactory. The anti-viral drug **amantadine** (Symmetrel) came into common use a few years ago. They all improve the rigidity, but have little effect on the tremor, and it is the tremor which often worries the patient more. Absolutely regular and adequate dosage is essential, but Parkinsonian patients rarely stick to one treatment for long and constantly complain of the side effects.

The treatment of Parkinsonism has been transformed in the last ten years or so by the use of the preparation **l-dopa.** This, when taken by mouth, is converted into **dopamine** in the brain and it is dopamine that is lacking in the basal nuclei of Parkinsonian patients. Its particular value is in the **akinetic** form of the disease, and the masking of the face disappears, the patient can get in and out of chairs more easily, stop, turn, accelerate, get out of baths, turn over in bed and generally quicken up in all movements. Tremor is much less responsive though on prolonged treatment this also improves. The drug does, however, have side-effects—nausea, indigestion and dizziness, but most serious is the production, on too high dosage, of **involuntary movements** of a different sort, almost choreo-athetosis (see p. 110) and usually referred to as **dyskinesia.** This can be stopped by reducing the dosage.

Most l-dopa taken by mouth is destroyed before it gets to the brain. The addition of **carbidopa** has prevented this to a large extent so that a combination of two drugs enables a much smaller dose of l-dopa to be equally effective. Unfortunately dyskinesia remains a major side-effect though some patients prefer this to the akinesia which incapacitated them previously.

The **tremor** has always been the most **resistant** symptom to medical treatment, and for this reason a variety of **surgical operations** have been devised, all of which have aimed at interrupting the extrapyramidal pathways. Of these by far the most effective has been the making, with great accuracy, of a small lesion in the part of the basal nuclei, usually the thalamus, without damaging the rest of the brain. This is a complex procedure called **stereotaxis.** Results vary, tremor and rigidity responding very much better than the other features of Parkinsonism and in properly selected cases may be very satisfactory. The ideal patient is one who has **unilateral** or predominantly unilateral tremor, preferably on the left side so that the lesion will be made in the **non-dominant hemisphere**; whose lips, chin and tongue are not affected; who shows no dementia; and who is in good general condition, under the age of 65 and not showing arterial degenerative disease. Bilateral operations are more inclined to be followed by disturbances of speech and memory and difficulty with urinary control. This danger is much reduced if a considerable interval is allowed to elapse between the two sides being done. However, the introduction of l-dopa has greatly reduced the number of stereotactic procedures that are required.

Other Involuntary Movements

Athetosis consists of **slow writhing** movements of the limbs, face and trunk, seen most frequently as a result of brain damage or anoxia at or before birth, and not necessarily developing for several years. It is one of the dangers of Rhesus incompatibility.

In **chorea** the movements are **very rapid,** each different from the next, accompanied by flapping of the tip of the protruded tongue; grimacing and respiratory irregularity. When both are present we speak of **choreo-athetosis.**

Classically chorea follows rheumatic fever (**Sydenham's chorea**) but this is now uncommon. It can occur in **pregnancy** and it is one of the rare complications of the use of **oral contraceptives.** A rather similar dyskinesia occurs in high doses of l-dopa.

Huntington's chorea is a strongly familial disease starting in middle life and accompanied by progressive mental deterioration.

Hemiballismus is a violent flaying movement of one arm and leg brought about by a vascular accident in a particular part of the brain called the **subthalamic nucleus.**

There is very little satisfactory treatment for athetosis but choreic movements can be substantially improved by the drug **tetrabenazine.** This is, therefore, useful in Huntington's and senile chorea but does not influence mental deterioration in the former.

Motor Neurone Disease

Degenerative changes may affect the motor system only—the **anterior horn cells,** the nuclei of some of the cranial nerves, and the fibres of the **pyramidal tracts.** This results in three syndromes—**progressive muscular atrophy, progressive bulbar palsy,** and **amyotrophic lateral sclerosis.** It is now realised that these are all part of the same disease, the difference in their signs depending upon which part of the motor system is most affected. They are, therefore, grouped together as motor neurone disease, the cause of which is unknown.

Symptoms

The disease most frequently develops between the ages of 40–60. **Weakness** may first be noticed in the hands, the shoulders, or the neck muscles. Occasionally the legs are first affected, usually as a painless footdrop. The hand and shoulder girdle muscles begin to waste, and gradually the weakness and **wasting** spreads throughout the body until the trunk muscles no longer give support, and weakness of the tongue and throat muscles makes **speech difficult,** and **swallowing** impossible. The term progressive bulbar palsy is used when these latter symptoms start the disease, and death may then occur before the rest of the body has become involved. In the variety called amyotrophic lateral sclerosis, pyramidal tract degeneration causes a spasticity which may predominate over wasting and weakness at first, but not for long.

Signs

Muscle **wasting** is usually first seen in the shoulder girdles and hands, where the weakness is often greater than the wasting might suggest. Later the wasting becomes widespread, and the **tongue** becomes small, wrinkled and paralysed. Bundles of muscle fibres show a constant jumping and flickering known as **fasciculation,** and this is clearly seen in the wasted tongue. Despite the wasting of the muscles, the tendon **reflexes** are greatly **exaggerated,** and it is this fact, combined with the fasciculation and normal sensation that gives the clue to the diagnosis.

Treatment

There is no effective treatment. The disease progresses inevitably to death, usually from respiratory infection, in from six months to two years, rarely longer.

Cerebral (Cortical) Atrophy

Atrophy, or shrinkage, of brain tissue may follow injury, inflammation or interference with blood supply, but the cells and fibres can also atrophy for reasons as yet unknown. As a result of loss of cerebral tissue, the **gyri** becomes **thinner,** the sulci wider and the **ventricles larger.** There are several different types of cerebral atrophy, of which the best known are called **Pick's disease** and **Alzheimer's disease.** Grouped together they are called the **presenile dementias.** In elderly patients, the blood supply to the brain is reduced due to arteriosclerotic narrowing of the arteries. Atrophy again results and this state is called senile dementia.

Symptoms

Memory is most noticeably disturbed. At first this is for recent events only, childhood being remembered clearly, but gradually all memory is lost, even of words spoken a few moments before. The patient becomes unable to look after the normal affairs of life, cannot be trusted to deal safely with money matters, or to cook. Later, assistance is required to dress and to find the way about the house. The physical state may remain good throughout, and the patient appear normal on casual meeting, but some are subject to recurrent fits.

Signs

The patients are **confused,** and **disorientated,** not knowing their own names, age, or those of their nearest relatives, not knowing where they are, nor the identity of those around them. Physical examination is usually normal.

Treatment

Fits must be controlled by anticonvulsants, and investigations must be carried out to make certain that the dementia is not due either to an operable cerebral tumour, Vitamin B.12 deficiency, folic acid deficiency or neurosyphilis. In general, though, these cases steadily deteriorate until they have no mind left, and need constant institutional care.

Normal Pressure Hydrocephalus

In this condition the symptoms previously mentioned are often associated with marked tremor and ataxia. They may follow a head injury or an intracranial haemorrhage. The **ventricles** are very **large** but there is **little** evidence of **cortical atrophy** when an air-encephalogram is carried out. It is thought that there is obstruction to absorption of C.S.F. and if a radioactive substance is introduced into the lumbar theca it will collect in the ventricle and fail to diffuse through the subarachnoid space. This can be measured by scanning (**the RISA scan**) or, if available, using metrizamide with the C.A.T scan, and some patients may be improved by the use of one of the **shunts** described on page 166. The results of this are not uniform but if successful can be very gratifying.

13 *TOXIC, METABOLIC, AND DEFICIENCY DISEASES*

Each of the diseases grouped together in this chapter is caused by (a) some **poison** acting on the nervous system, (b) a **shortage** of some substance which is essential for nervous tissue to function correctly, or (c) both. The poison (**toxin**) may be produced by abnormalities inside the body, as, for instance, in uraemia, or it may be taken in from outside, as in drug addiction. A vital substance may become deficient because not enough is taken in, as in starvation, because it is not absorbed properly, as in pernicious anaemia, or because the body fails to use it properly once it is absorbed.

The **peripheral nerves** and **posterior columns** of the cord appear to be particularly vulnerable to chronic toxic and deficiency states, and before passing on to some of the more common diseases, some general remarks are made about the terms polyneuritis and polyneuropathy.

Polyneuritis and Polyneuropathy

Strictly speaking, **neuritis** means inflammation of a nerve, and **polyneuritis** inflammation of many nerves. Nerves do not, however, often become inflamed in the true sense of the word, and many physicians prefer the term **polyneuropathy.** When a word ends in '-opathy' it means there is something wrong, but it is not an inflammation, and *exactly* what it is may not be certain. The same ending is used in encephalopathy, myelopathy, etc.

In a polyneuritis or polyneuropathy the symptoms usually start in the fingers and hands, toes and feet on both sides—hence the alternative term peripheral neuritis. They can consist of **numbness, pins and needles,** or **burning**; or they can be mainly motor, consisting of **weakness** and later **wasting.** They are usually both sensory and motor. These symptoms spread upwards to involve the calves, thigh and hip muscles, and the arms and shoulder girdles, and in severe cases, may even affect the trunk, respiratory and facial muscles. The **reflexes** are characteristically **absent,** and there is **loss of sensation** in the hands and forearms, and the feet and lower legs (**glove and stocking anaesthesia**). The condition may range from mild tinglings in all four limbs, to total paralysis of all muscles, the patient requiring tracheostomy and an artificial respirator. The absence of signs of meningeal irritation, the rather slower onset, the symmetry of the paralysis and the presence of sensory loss distinguishes polyneuritis from poliomyelitis.

The exact cause of many cases of polyneuropathy is never discovered, but fortunately recovery is very common. Polyneuritic signs will repeatedly be mentioned in this chapter, but it is convenient to describe one well-known syndrome first, though it may not be of toxic or metabolic origin.

Acute 'Infective' Polyneuritis

This disease develops rapidly, often a few weeks after a vague pyrexial illness, and sometimes as a complication of known infections such as glandular fever. The symptoms are those of a polyneuritis, but the motor paralysis can become very severe, and it is very characteristic for there to be **bilateral facial paralysis.** The muscles are very tender, but sensory loss is often relatively slight. The diagnosis is confirmed by finding a very **high protein** in the C.S.F (often over 250 mg/100 ml), but no rise in cells. After two or three weeks of great disability the patient slowly improves and usually makes a complete recovery. This probably represents one of the auto-immune diseases where the patient's own body defences react to damage to its own tissue. Along with other such disorders, **A.C.T.H.** or cortisone given in the acute stage may speed up the recovery, but given later is of little use. This condition is also named the **Guillain-Barré syndrome,** after the two French neurologists who described it during the first World War.

Most other polyneuropathies are similar as regards symptoms and signs, but develop more slowly, the face is usually not affected, and the C.S.F. protein is rarely so high.

DEFICIENCY DISEASES

Subacute Combined Degeneration

This condition is normally associated with **pernicious anaemia,** the underlying cause of each being atrophy of the mucous membrane of the stomach. As a result, factors for the development of red blood cells, and for the nutrition of nervous tissue, are not absorbed from the food. The vital substance **deficient** has been isolated from the liver and is called **Vitamin B.12,** and in its absence the number of red cells which develops is small, but they are larger and carry more haemoglobin than usual (**macrocytic anaemia**). The deficiency also results in a gradual **degeneration** of the **posterior columns** and **pyramidal traacts** in the spinal cord, together with a polyneuropathy—hence the term 'subacute combined'.

The patients, usually middle-aged and white-haired, often women, complain of **numbness** and **tingling** in the fingers and toes, soreness of the calves (due to peripheral neuritis) and **unsteadiness** in walking, especially in the dark (due to posterior column degeneration). On questioning, they admit to soreness of the **tongue.**

If the patient has had no treatment there is a mild pallor, with a slightly yellowish tinge. The tongue is shiny and sore (superficial glossitis). The limbs are weak and the reflexes may be absent (if polyneuritis predominates), or exaggerated (if pyramidal tract degeneration predominates). The plantar reflexes are, however, usually extensor. Position sense and vibration sense are impaired in the legs and there is a **postural ataxia** (see p. 32). The **calves** are **tender** and there may be slight impairment of sensation of glove and stocking distribution.

The blood count and sternal marrow show the characteristics of pernicious anaemia, providing no treatment has been given. Owing to the atrophy of the stomach hydrochloric acid is not secreted, so that a **fractional test meal** shows no free acid even after the injection of histamine (**a histamine-fast achlorhydria**). The serum Vitamin B.12 level is very low (if untreated). The C.S.F. is normal.

Vitamin B.12 is given by injection. Quite a small dose corrects the anaemia, but to treat the neurological lesion much higher doses are required. 250 µg should be given daily at first, then once or twice weekly for many months and less frequently permanently. The polyneuritic features should clear up, but the symptoms of spinal cord disease, if present for a very long time, may only partly recover. Relapse is always possible if treatment is inadequate.

Other Vitamin B.12 Deficiency Syndromes

Absorption of B.12 may be defective in a variety of intestinal diseases. **Steatorrhoea,** where the absorption of fat is deficient; **surgical** removal of the stomach; **Crohn's disease; chronic diarrhoea,** are a few examples. In these there are deficiencies of other vitamins as well, such as Vitamin B.1, pyridoxine, nicotinic acid and folic acid. The symptoms and signs may be suggestive of polyneuritis or of subacute combined degeneration, but they are not associated with a histamine-fast achlorhydria, or the typical bone marrow of pernicious anaemia.

Vitamin B.1 Deficiency

In states of starvation, inadequate diet or severe gastric disturbance (e.g. **alcoholic gastritis**), not enough **Vitamin B.1** (thiamine) may be absorbed, and a polyneuritis can result. In severe cases the heart enlarges and fails, and oedema of the limbs develops. The condition is then called **Beri-beri.** Treatment is to give large doses of **thiamine** by injection (100 mg daily). Changes may take place in the upper brain stem, causing paralysis of eye movement, ataxia, confusion and even coma. This is called **Wernicke's encephalopathy.** Treatment, usually effective, consists of large doses of **thiamine** by injection (100 mg daily).

Nicotinic Acid Deficiency

If **nicotinic acid,** another of the B. group of vitamins, is deficient, **pellagra** develops. The nervous symptoms may be those of a polyneuropathy, or a syndrome similar to subacute combined degeneration, but in addition there is a scaly brown **rash** on those parts of the skin exposed to **light.**

Folic Acid Deficiency

Folic acid is also concerned in blood formation, and deficiency causes not only anaemia, but **polyneuropathy,** and in some cases severe **mental changes** which can be cured by by restoring the blood folate level. The cause of low serum folate levels is often obscure, but one known cause is the prolonged use of high doses of anticonvulsants. This must be remembered and corrected if anaemia and mental changes develop in chronic epileptics.

NEUROLOGICAL COMPLICATIONS OF CERTAIN METABOLIC DISEASES

Diabetes

Polyneuritis is a common complication of poorly controlled diabetes. The symptoms are particularly sensory, with severe burning sensations in the hands and feet, numbness of the extremities and increasing difficulty in walking. The exact cause is still rather uncertain, and though vitamins are usually given, it does not respond well to treatment. Complete control of the diabetes is essential to prevent worsening.

There is always danger of **diabetic coma** in poorly controlled patients. Usually there is general malaise for some hours or days, the patient becomes increasingly thirsty, then starts **frequent vomiting** and soon becomes **dehydrated** and **drowsy,** passing into coma if not treated. If there is some additional infection, such as a **carbuncle,** even a well controlled diabetic may go into coma. Control breaks down, the urine is loaded with sugar and acetone, and the blood sugar is very high. The treatment required is **insulin,** probably given **intravenously,** balanced with **intravenous glucose,** together with saline to correct the dehydration.

Hypoglycaemic Coma

In contrast, if the **blood sugar** falls **too low,** the patient goes into **hypoglycaemic coma.** A diabetic receiving insulin starts **sweating** profusely shortly after one of his usual doses, then becomes **ataxic, confused,** may have **convulsions,** and loses consciousness. The blood sugar is very low. This state can be corrected rapidly by giving **sugar** by mouth, or intravenously, or by giving an injection of **adrenaline,** which causes sugar to pour into the blood from the liver. Prolonged hypoglycaemia may cause permanent brain damage so that early recognition and correction of these symptoms is vital.

Spontaneous Hypoglycaemia

Very low blood sugar may sometimes occur in people who are not taking insulin. The results vary from transient disturbances of behaviour, episodes of ataxia and drowsiness, to fits and loss of consciousness, almost always with profuse sweating. The most common cause is that a **small tumour** has formed of cells in the pancreas which secrete insulin—**the Islets of Langerhans.** The condition can be diagnosed by starving the patient for 24 hours or more. The blood sugar will then fall below 40 mg per 100 ml, some of the symptoms described develop, and if an **E.E.G.** (p. 177) is taken at the same time, it will show **gross abnormality.** The diagnosis can be confirmed by giving glucose by mouth or injection, for the clinical state, the blood sugar and the E.E.G. will be returned to normal within 15 minutes. In such a case a surgeon will explore the pancreas and removal of the islet-cell tumour will cure the condition.

Potassium Deficiency

If the blood potassium falls **very low** a weakness of the limbs can develop amounting to total **flaccid paralysis.** Power will be restored to normal by giving potassium chloride or citrate. A low level such as this may occur in patients on cortisone and in some forms of nephritis when the potassium is excreted in excess. The same paralysis may develop spontaneously, however, in cases of **familial periodic paralysis.** It occurs repeatedly while the patient is asleep, especially if following a very heavy meal. Several members of a family are affected, and the attacks can be reduced in severity by taking potassium regularly by mouth. During **renal dialysis** there are many possible disturbances of blood chemistry. These include the potassium, and signs such as these need to be carefully noted.

Carcinomatous Neuropathy

A slow **degenerative** process of the **sensory fibres** in the peripheral nerves and the posterior columns can occur in patients who have a carcinoma of the **bronchus,** and occasionally with other carcinomas. These patients develop progressive numbness, weakness and wasting of the legs, with increasing ataxia due to loss of position sense, and these symptoms may be present long before the carcinoma itself is discovered. Death from general weakness may occur, the tumour not being discovered until autopsy. The explanation is unknown; it is not due to metastases, but treatment is usually of no avail. Very occasionally successful removal of the primary tumour is followed by recovery. A similarly mysterious degeneration of the cerebellum, producing a cerebellar ataxia, sometimes occurs in patients with unsuspected carcinoma. Again the bronchus is the most common site, but in women ovarian tumours may be responsible.

Some think tumours secrete a substance which renders vitamins inactive at the nerve endings, but this is not proven and high dosage of vitamins gives very variable results.

INBORN ERRORS OF METABOLISM

Some people are born with a tendency for one of the vital chemical processes of the body to go wrong. As a result some substance, which is normally broken down and excreted, builds up in the body to toxic proportions. There are many such diseases, all very rare, a few of which affect the nervous system.

Wilson's Disease (hepato-lenticular degeneration) is due to a deficiency of a substance called coeruloplasmin, which normally carries copper in the blood. As a result the level of **copper** cannot be maintained in the blood, excessive amounts are lost in the urine and, more important, are deposited in various organs, including the liver and the basal ganglia (lenticular nucleus). Several members of a family are affected. Severe **involuntary movements** develop in youth and the patients become progressively more disabled and **deteriorate mentally.** Later they develop **liver failure.** Copper is also deposited in the corneas of the eyes, producing a golden brown ring—**the Kayser-Fleischer ring**—which is quite diagnostic. Treatment is by **penicillamine.** This substance extracts the copper from the brain, and increases its excretion in the urine. There is a striking improvement in the patient's clinical condition, which appears to be maintained for many years in early cases.

Porphyria (haematoporphyrinuria). Porphyrins are substances concerned in the formation of **blood pigments.** Sometimes metabolism of these substances is disturbed and large amounts are excreted in the urine, where they can be detected. In some cases they cause it to turn a **port wine colour** after exposure to light. In others special tests are necessary. The skin of some patients **blisters** easily on exposure to sunlight. Others have attacks of **abdominal pain** and **mental disturbance** lasting several weeks, during which time they develop a **polyneuritis.** These attacks recover spontaneously and are particularly liable to follow administration of barbiturates. No treatment is known.

Phenylketonuric Oligophrenia. In a very small percentage of mentally deficient infants, abnormal substances called phenylketones are excreted in the urine, due to a defect in the metabolism of an amino acid called phenylalanine. They can be detected by adding a few drops of **ferric chloride** to the urine, a test which can easily be carried out on the baby's **nappies.** A special diet free from phenylalanine has been used with considerable benefit, and the condition is important in being about the only type of mental deficiency which is preventable.

TOXIC DISEASES

Alcoholism

When a person is drunk he develops a disturbance of co-ordination. This results in double vision, slurring of speech (dysarthria), unsteadiness of the arms and legs, and ataxia of gait. These develop during a bout of drinking and clear up some hours afterwards (usually with a hangover!). If excessive alcohol is taken over a long period of time, however, the effects differ. The toxin acts directly on the **brain** and **liver,** and also causes sufficient damage to the **stomach** to prevent the absorption of vitamins, especially **Vitamin B.1.** The direct effects consist of gross **tremulousness** of the whole body, followed a few days later by wild **confusion** and agitation with terrifying visual and auditory **hallucinations,** and absolute wakefulness. This is the famous **delirium tremens (D.Ts.),** and occurs in chronic alcoholics who have had a heavy bout of drinking and then stopped. Treatment is by **sedation,** and *not* by giving more alcohol, though this practice dies hard.

After years of heavy drinking, the deficiency of Vitamin B.1 causes severe damage to the **brain stem.** This results in mental confusion, paralysis of eye movements, double vision, ataxia of arms and legs, and in addition a polyneuropathy (i.e. the condition called **Wernicke's encephalopathy**) and must be treated urgently with massive doses of Vitamin B.1.

Alcoholic polyneuritis is not uncommon in all chronic alcoholics and responds to vitamin therapy provided the alcohol is avoided *completely*. Half measures are of no use. Unhappily very few true chronic alcoholics ever succeed in complete abstention.

Barbiturates and Anti-epileptic Drugs

If an enormous dose of barbiturates (e.g. phenobarbitone) is suddenly taken, as, for instance, in an **attempted suicide, coma** develops rapidly, with complete **flaccidity** of the limbs, absent reflexes and often **collapse** of the circulation. The patient can only be saved if the **stomach** is washed out at once, and intravenous **cerebral stimulants** such as megamide given until there are signs of arousal. Excessive amounts of this drug taken over a long period of time produce slurring of speech, ataxia of the limbs and recurrent drowsiness.

Many poorly controlled epileptics develop toxic effects from combinations of too much phenobarbitone, epanutin and mysoline. They also develop **drowsiness,** gross **ataxia, nystagmus,** and **dysarthria,** but often with sufficient headache and vomiting to raise suspicions of a cerebellar tumour.

Folic acid Deficiency also can occur after prolonged heavy dosage. Modern methods of estimating the levels of many of the anticonvulsants in the blood help to prevent these effects and have also shown that certain drugs interact with each other to produce too high a level of one or other in the blood, e.g. sulthiame and phenytoin. Others may reduce each others' effectiveness.

The problem of treatment is that if anticonvulsants are stopped suddenly **status epilepticus** may occur, so that, though reduction is essential, it must always be gradual and carried out under conditions where treatment is readily available if a series of fits develop (see p. 142).

Miscellaneous Drugs

Tranquillisers even in moderate doses may cause slowing of reactions, defective judgement and slight unsteadiness, while if combined with alcohol these signs can become very marked. Diazepam can cause a fall of blood pressure on standing up (postural hypotension) and so result in fainting. Very large doses of tranquillisers taken over a long period produce a syndrome almost indistinguishable from **Parkinsonism** (see p. 107).

Amphetamine (and to a lesser extent **belladonna**) causes excitement, agitation, tremor, rapid pulse, collapse and delirium. **Belladonna** or **atropine** also causes dilation of the pupils. (Probably the commonest cause of a fixed dilated pupil in an otherwise perfectly healthy nurse is that she has accidentally rubbed some atropine in her eye.)

Lead produces a **polyneuropathy,** especially wrist drop, while the type of lead used in some paints and petrols can cause a cerebral disturbance called lead **encephalopathy,** with headache, mental change, fits and even coma. Infants can get lead poisoning from sucking toys painted with lead-containing paints.

Mercury Poisoning is rarely a problem these days though when used in the hat-making industry it used to cause tremors and ataxia known as Hatters' Shakes. Some plant sprays contains a form of mercury which if inhaled can cause postural ataxia. In some countries waste products containing mercury discharged into rivers polluted the fish. When these were caught and eaten the local people (and their cats, but not their dogs) developed a syndrome very like an acute attack of disseminated sclerosis.

Arsenic taken for long periods by mouth can cause a polyneuropathy and a type that used to be given intravenously in the treatment of syphilis caused an encephalopathy.

Treatment of Malignancy. Certain of the drugs used (e.g. vincristine) cause polyneuropathy and others used in leukaemia (e.g. methotrexate) can cause a severe encephalopathy.

Chloroquin, used in the treatment of rheumatoid arthritis (and malaria) can cause retinal damage and visual field defects.

Enterovioform, popular against travellers' diarrhoea, can, in susceptible people, produce a neurological disturbance very like an acute episode of disseminated sclerosis.

Bush Tea. Certain types of this tea, popular in the West Indies can cause a spastic ataxia also resembling disseminated sclerosis (though it is not the usual cause of the West Indian spastic paraplegia).

Oral Contraceptives can cause **cerebral thrombosis, papilloedema, chorea,** an increase in **migraine** and perhaps in **epilepsy.** These are dealt with in the appropriate chapters.

Most of these toxic effects can be cured providing the substance is withdrawn absolutely, but if intoxication has been present for a very long time, permanent damage may have taken place in the nervous system, and cure may not be complete. This particularly applies to drug and alcohol addiction, for, in addition, one can never be certain that the patient is not still secretly obtaining supplies, and in order to do this they show fantastic ingenuity and complete disregard either for the truth, or for the obvious consequences of their actions.

One of the serious facts realised by the profession in recent years is how many strange syndromes can be **iatrogenic,** i.e. produced by doctors, or rather by the treatment that they have ordered. Ever since the thalidomide tragedy a national committee now called the Committee for the Safety of Medicines has been examining all reported toxic effects of drugs, and looking into the safety of any new drug before it is marketed to prevent similar catastrophes occurring, and to give the profession early warning of any unexpected side-effects consistently reported to them.

14 *HEREDITARY AND FAMILIAL DISEASES*

A **hereditary** disease is one which is passed on from generation to generation; **familial** disease affects several members of the same family. Most conditions coming under this heading show both these features and the term **'heredo-familial'** is therefore commonly used. The so-called heredo-familial diseases of the nervous system are those which can be traced in several relatives, though the relationship may sometimes be a distant one, and careful enquiry into the family history is essential. Examples have already been described, e.g. Wilson's disease, periodic paralysis; others will be dealt with later, e.g. epilepsy, muscular dystrophy. When using the term, however, most neurologists are referring to the group of uncommon diseases described in this chapter, which are degenerative in type, and tend to produce abnormalities either of co-ordination, or of the peripheral nerves.

THE HEREDO-FAMILIAL ATAXIAS

This is a group of diseases in which several members of a family develop a **progressive ataxia.** In any particular family the symptoms and signs are much the same, but in different families they vary, mainly in the age at which the trouble starts and what parts of the nervous system are mainly affected. As a result these diseases have been given various names, after the physicians who first described them, e.g. **Marie's ataxia, Sanger-Brown's ataxia.** The differences are not of great practical importance, however, and certain features commonly occur in all.

Symptoms

Increasing clumsiness and unsteadiness of the arms and legs develop and may quickly be recognised by the patients as the symptoms suffered by (say) their father or brother. There may also be defective vision and difficulty in speech, but there is no headache, vomiting, vertigo, or diplopia as in posterior fossa tumour, and the condition advances steadily and not by remissions and relapses, as in disseminated sclerosis.

Signs

The main sign is ataxia. This is due to cerebellar disease, with slurring of speech, nystagmus, and unsteadiness of the arms, legs and gait. The tendon reflexes are usually absent, but as the pyramidal tracts are affected in some cases, there may be extensor plantar responses. **Pes cavus** is common, and often is also found in relatives who are otherwise unaffected. **Optic atrophy** is often found on examination, but the patients rarely complain of loss of vision.

Some Special Varieties

Friedreich's Ataxia develops in adolesence. It shows, in addition to optic atrophy, nystagmus, absent reflexes, extensor plantars and pes cavus, marked loss of position and vibration sense, with a postural ataxia, due to degeneration of the posterior columns. The back muscles are weak and severe scoliosis is common. The heart muscle may be affected and many patients die from heart failure.

In **Olivo-ponto-cerebellar Degeneration,** which develops in middle life, **dysarthria** is a major symptom, and as well as the cerebellar ataxia, there is spasticity and exaggeration of the reflexes. This condition often resembles disseminated sclerosis, but it advances without remissions, is often familial, and the dysarthria is outstanding.

Hereditary Spastic Paraplegia is distinct from the others, for cerebellar signs are absent. The legs become progressively more **spastic** in early middle age, and the gait becomes 'scissors-like'. There is gross exaggeration of reflexes and extensor plantars, but no true ataxia. The feet again show a deformity similar to **pes cavus.**

THE HEREDITARY NEUROPATHIES

Another group of rare diseases is caused by degeneration of the peripheral nerves, in some mainly of motor fibres, in others mainly of sensory fibres.

Peroneal Muscular Atrophy (or Charcot-Marie-Tooth's disease). This is a neuropathy, not purely a degeneration of muscle, as was once thought and as the name suggests. It affects either sex but is much more common in males and develops in adolescence or early adult life.

Symptoms

Walking becomes increasingly difficult for the legs have to be lifted unusually high to avoid catching the toes. Wasting is first noted in the legs and later in the hands and forearms.

Signs

There is a high-stepping gait due to **bilateral foot drop,** each foot being slapped down in turn. There is pes cavus, and the feet and hands are blue and cold. The wasting is the most characteristic feature (Fig. 14.1) because, though very marked, it stops suddenly **halfway up** the thighs and forearms. The shoulder girdles, upper arms, hip girdles and upper thighs are normal, making the legs look like inverted bottles. There is a little glove and stocking sensory loss (see p. 33), and vibration sense is impaired. All tendon reflexes are absent. The condition progresses very slowly without causing incapacity until late in life.

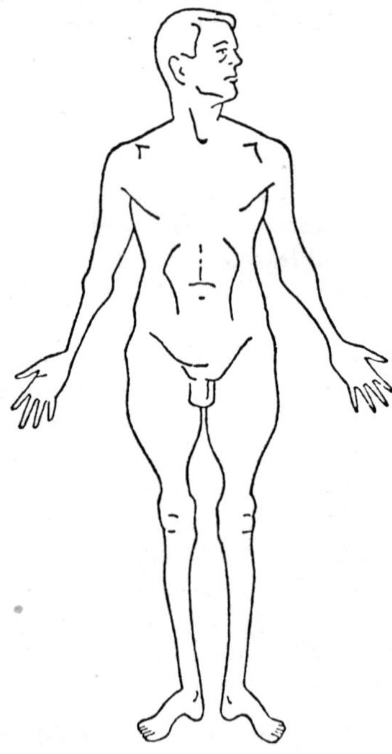

FIG. 14.1 Sketch of a case of peroneal muscular atrophy. Note that the wasting appears to stop suddenly at mid-forearm and mid-thigh.

Hypertrophic Polyneuritis. This disease has all the features of a polyneuritis (p. 114), but it progresses slowly over many years. It can give a picture similar to peroneal muscular atrophy, but there is great **thickening** of the **peripheral nerves,** which can be felt at the elbows, below the knees and on the dorsum of the feet.

Hereditary Sensory Neuropathy. In this it is sensation that is severely impaired, so that painless infected sores develop on the fingers and toes, which may have to be amputated, or which drop off by themselves as in leprosy.

It is not uncommon to find examples of more than one of these diseases in the same family, and indeed sometimes there appear to be two types in the same patient. It seems that they may all, in some way, be linked together. It is also very common, on examining the relatives, to find unmistakeable signs in someone who is entirely symptom-free. These are called **'formes frustes'** of the disease.

They all progress slowly and no drug therapy is available. Physiotherapy aimed at educating the patient to co-ordinate his movements, can make considerable, if temporary, improvement. Sooner or later, however, disability becomes severe, though only comparatively rarely do these patients become bedridden.

A lot more is known about the inheritance of these diseases now and it is often necessary to give advice to prospective parents regarding possible danger of their children becoming affected—this must be well-informed advice.

THE LEUCODYSTROPHIES

There are several diseases affecting children, which may be familial, in which degenerative changes occur particularly in the **white matter** of the brain. These appear in early childhood and may cause successive children in a family to become increasingly backward, ataxic, to develop fits, weakness of the limbs progressing finally to complete paralysis and loss of intellect. Best known is the **metachromatic leucodystrophy,** which can be diagnosed in life by finding substances called **sulphatides** in the urine, or in biopsies of kidney, peripheral nerve or brain. No method of halting the disease is known. Others in this group are less common, all are rare, and many only diagnosed after death.

15 *DISORDERS OF FUNCTION; MIGRAINE, NEURALGIAS, VERTIGO*

The diseases so far described have all been due to some abnormality of the structure of the nervous system. In the course of everyday life, however, most people who have symptoms which might be related to the nervous system do not have anything wrong with the way it is made, but with the way it works (or functions). Common symptoms such as headache and giddiness fall into this group. Unfortunately, the term 'functional' is often used to suggest an imaginary disturbance, because, of course, psychological upsets disturb function, rather than structure. There are, however, many disorders of the normal functioning of the brain, its blood vessels, and its coverings, which produce vivid symptoms, the reason for which may not be known, or which may indeed have a psychological *basis*, but there is no doubt that they are real.

Rather surprisingly, the skull and the brain are not capable of feeling pain. This is why brain surgery can be done under local anaesthesia and in some countries often is. It is from the scalp, its muscles and blood vessels, and from the dura, its venous sinuses, and the blood vessels at the base of the brain that pain can arise. Of these, headache most commonly originates in the muscles, the blood vessels, and the dura, and it is produced by tension in, or stretching of, these structures.

MIGRAINE

Mee-graine (not my-graine) is due to a disturbance in the behaviour of the cranial blood vessels. Exactly what causes an attack is not known and there may be many causes, but it seems certain that chemical changes in and around the blood vessel walls play an important role in causation. It is generally believed that symptoms are produced by **spasm** of vessels inside the skull, and **dilatation** of vessels outside the skull, the spasm producing the warning of an attack (the **aura**) and the dilatation producing the **headache.** One can argue for and against this theory.

Migrainous attacks sometimes bear an obvious relationship to such things as menstruation, anxiety, or excitement, but others come apparently out of the blue, often occurring at weekends. Some foods are liable to produce attacks, chocolate being the most common. They usually start in youth, sometimes in childhood, affect women more than men, and are common in perfectionists who hold difficult, responsible, frustrating posts, and live at high pressure. It is strongly hereditary, and allergic disorders (asthma, eczema) may be found in the same family.

Symptoms

The Aura. The first symptoms depend on which blood vessels go into 'spasm'. Not all attacks have a clear aura, but many episodes begin with flashing, scintillating **lights** zig-zagging across the visual fields, and sometimes forming coloured patterns with a dark centre and jagged edges. These are called **teichopsia** and **fortification spectra.** Other visual auras include loss of **half** of the **visual field** (homonymous hemianopia); of the outer fields of each eye (bitemporal hemianopia); or complete loss in both eyes, or small patches of loss in both eyes (**scotomata**). These symptoms are due to spasm affecting vessels supplying the optic nerves, the chiasma, or the occipital visual cortex. If the middle cerebral artery is involved the patient develops **numbness** of one hand and arm, one half of the face and tongue, and even **dysphasia.** If the basilar artery is involved there may be bilateral blindness, vertigo, tinnitus, tingling in both hands and legs, and dysarthria.

Any of these symptoms (which may be very alarming) last from a few minutes to as long as an hour, then they die away, to be replaced by the headache.

The Headache. Migraine headache is said to be one-sided, but quite as often it affects the whole head, or purely the occipital region. It is due to dilatation of the superficial arteries, so that it **throbs** violently and the superficial temporal vessel may be seen to stand out. It increases to a maximum when **vomiting** occurs, and there is then improvement, the patient goes to sleep, and probably wakes free from pain. A migrainous headache occasionally may last 24–48 hours, and vomiting is sometimes constant and prolonged. *Very* occasionally, just at the stage when the aura changes to the headache, the patient may lose consciousness for a few moments.

Treatment

Once the headache has started, there is nothing more likely to influence it than the **aspirin**-containing analgesics, but the vomiting may prevent their usefulness. Effervescent preparations of paracetamol, (e.g. paragesic) are superior to others, but their absorption from the stomach is retarded during a migrainous attack. This can be overcome to a large extent by giving **metaclopramide** (maxolon) 10 minutes beforehand.

If there is a long aura, however, **ergotamine preparations,** taken early, may prevent the headache from developing. By mouth they are not very effective, though cafergot in tablets allowed to dissolve under the tongue, or used in **suppositories,** does help some people. Ergotamine tartrate by **injection** is the most satisfactory. This may make some patients sick and should be preceded by **Largactil** or **Dramamine.** Ergotamine inhalers were hoped to give good results but their dosage is unreliable and too frequent use can lead to overdosage. In fact, long term ergotamine administration produces a condition of **mild toxicity** with malaise and chronic headache often mistaken for the migraine itself. The aura may also be very short or absent. In such cases long term prevention should be attempted.

Quite regular sedation by **prochlorperazine** (Stemetil) or **diazepam** (Valium) can be valuable in cases of moderate severity, while intractable cases, which really are genuine migraine (and not simply tension headaches) may respond to **methysergide** (Deseril). This drug is very effective, but it must be taken for no more than three months without a break of a month or six weeks, to avoid undesirable side-effects. Recently **pizotofen** (Sanomigran) has been introduced for similar cases and has less toxicity if rather less beneficial effect.

There is no wonder cure, however, though there are plenty claimed, some of which border on frank charlatanry. It is said that migraine sufferers should be protected from the strains and stresses of life, for these help to stimulate attacks. The idea, however, is a bad one. They will be happier, healthier, more useful individuals if they accept their tendency to headaches and carry on their normal lives, which they usually do efficiently. The attacks tend to subside as patients get older and many women cease to have trouble after the menopause. In others however the development of hypertension worsens and prolongs the attacks.

A patient's views as to what brings on or prevents attacks should not be dismissed too lightly. If he has found that pickles taken on a cream bun at 11 o'clock every night will prevent his attacks, it is, after all, his headache, and he should know.

Ophthalmoplegic Migraine

Severe pain over one eye, similar to migraine, may sometimes be followed by double vision, **ptosis** and **paralysis** of the **IIIrd nerve** which lasts a week or more. In adults the majority of these cases are due, not to migraine, but to pressure on the IIIrd nerve by an aneurysm on the Circle of Willis. In childhood, however, usually in boys and despite careful arteriography, no abnormality may be found, and for want of a better term the name is retained.

Familial Hemiplegic Migraine

Numbness of one half of the body may occur in ordinary migraine, but sometimes there is frank **paralysis** of one arm and leg, lasting several days after 24–48 hours of headache. The mechanism is obscure, and this diagnosis can only be made if other members of the same family have identical attacks because this syndrome, in isolation, is much more likely to be due to a small bleed from a vascular anomaly (angioma or aneurysm).

Cough Headache

Cough headache is due to vascular distension during the act of coughing. Very severe pain develops either over one eye or in the head generally, lasting some moments after the coughing ceases. This is frightening, but not serious and the attacks usually stop after several months.

Periodic Migrainous Neuralgia

Migraine rarely disturbs a patient's sleep. Migrainous neuralgia almost always does. The attacks occur every night at about **2–3 a.m.,** for weeks on end, followed by months or years of freedom. The pain is always behind the same eye, and is accompanied by **reddening** and **running** of the eye, blocking of that side of the nose and flushing of that side of the face. It lasts ½–2 hours and is very severe. Attacks may also occur in the daytime, often at exactly the same time each day.

During a bout, an **injection** of **ergotamine tartrate** last thing at night, given by the patient himself much as a diabetic gives himself insulin, will stop the majority of attacks. This condition is sometimes called **histamine cephalgia,** or **cluster headaches.**

Muscle Tension Headache

This is the most common of all headaches and is, if the truth were told, the type of headache that most people who have diagnosed themselves as suffering from migraine actually have. Everyone gets 'tensed up' at some time or another. In some this **tension** affects the **scalp muscles** resulting in a headache that is much more prolonged than migraine, lasting days or weeks, often described as 'a pressure', or a 'tight band round the head and down the neck'. There is no aura, vomiting or disturbance of sleep. Some patients say they have never had a day free from headache for 10–20 years. The patients need not themselves be tense, but though they complain bitterly it is equally obvious that they are not ill. Frank explanation of the cause of the headache, combined with regular doses of prochlorperazine (Stemetil) or diazepam (Valium) help many sufferers and as there is an element of **depression** in almost all cases small regular doses of an antidepressant can be of additional help.

NEURALGIAS

Strictly speaking, neuralgia is pain in the distribution of a nerve. The term is often used rather vaguely. Some recurring severe pains, however, fall into a definite pattern which can be recognised and separated from others.

Trigeminal Neuralgia (tic douloureux)

This is an intense spasmodic pain affecting the area supplied by one of the branches of the Vth cranial nerve. It may affect all ages, but is less common below the age of 50.

Symptoms

Intense **stabs** of pain, each lasting only a few **seconds,** but often frequently repeated, shoot upwards from the upper lip, or upwards from the eyebrows, or downwards into the point of the jaw and the side of the tongue. They may always start from one **'trigger' point,** and can be brought on by touching this point, washing the face, shaving, exposure to cold winds, eating, drinking, or even talking. The face is contorted during an attack, but between attacks the patient is free of pain.

Treatment

The trigeminal nerve can either be **injected** with alcohol, or the nerve root **divided** by an intracranial operation. Both leave that side of the face numb, but following the injection there are often troublesome tinglings of which the patients complain bitterly.

A drug, **carbamazepine** (Tegretol) has recently been found to suppress the pain, if taken regularly, in the majority of patients. In many however the pain eventually breaks through, and surgery becomes necessary. **Spontaneous remissions** are common however, and drug therapy may tide the patient over until a remission occurs, which may last for years.

Atypical Facial Neuralgia

Many patients, usually women, complain of a **constant burning** pain, lasting for months or years, affecting one part of the face, but often spreading a little to the other side. They often date its onset from some dental treatment, say it is severe enough to contemplate suicide, but never seem to be any real discomfort. They are **depressed** and there is usually some serious deficiency in their lives, e.g. loss of their husband, or a failure to have children, and it is as if concentration on this pain in some way fills this gap. Treatment is exceedingly unsatisfactory, and drug addiction is a constant danger.

Post-herpetic Neuralgia

After an attack of **herpes zoster** (p. 76) neuralgic pain may persist for months or years. This is rare in the young, but common in the aged, especially affecting those who have had **ophthalmic herpes,** i.e. herpes of the 1st division of the Vth nerve. Like atypical facial neuralgia, despite their complaints the patients never seem to be in pain; the pain appears to become part of their personality and to govern their lives, and those of their near relatives. Even nerve root section does not successfully cure it, all forms of medical treatment fail, and there is danger of drug addiction.

VERTIGO

A patient who has vertigo feels that her or his surroundings are **spinning** round, either horizontally or vertically. A complaint of 'giddiness' may or may not mean vertigo, for the word is often clumsily used for a sense of instability, or attacks of faintness.

True vertigo is due to a disturbance of the **vestibular** system, which consists of the semicircular canals in the inner ear (the labyrinth), the vestibular branch of the VIIIth nerve and its nuclei in the brain stem, and the fibres which pass from these to the cerebellum, the temporal lobes and the spinal cord. Obviously, it is a very complicated mechanism and lesions producing vertigo may occur at many sites. The most common site, however, is in the **semicircular canals.**

Acute Labyrinthitis

This term is often used, but it is doubtful if the condition really exists, i.e. as a true inflammation of the semicircular canals. The symptoms start suddenly with severe **vertigo, vomiting** and

unsteadiness, but no deafness. They last a few days, and then clear up spontaneously. The patient is kept at strict rest, given one of the chlorpromazine (Largactil) or dimenhydrinate (Dramamine) group of drugs, and then mobilised only very gradually. This syndrome sometimes occurs in epidemics, which suggests an infective cause.

Ménière's Disease

For reasons unknown part of the labyrinth sometimes becomes swollen and this produces a fairly characteristic sequence of events.

Symptoms

The patient is prone to **sudden attacks** of vertigo, often severe enough to fling him to the ground. During the attack, which lasts several hours, the patient **vomits** repeatedly and is too unsteady to stand. In between attacks **tinnitus** develops in one ear, followed by gradually increasing **deafness.** Finally, the other ear may be similarly involved. Eventually the vertigo stops, leaving severe deafness.

Signs

Nystagmus and **unsteadiness** are present during an attack, and the patients lie flat, not daring to move. In between attacks an increasing **nerve deafness** in one or other ear is the only sign.

Treatment

Dramamine or Largactil should be given by injection in an acute attack, and taken regularly by mouth in between times. In severe cases a decompression or destruction of the labyrinth may be carried out, or the VIIIth nerve may be divided. Patients need to be grossly disabled by the attacks before this is recommended, for a sense of instability may be very troublesome afterwards, and more recently ultrasonic waves have been used to make similar lesions.

Arteriosclerotic Vertigo

In elderly people with **atheroma** of the vertebral and basilar arteries, sudden attacks of vertigo on movement are common. If small vessels supplying the vestibular system become blocked severe vertigo may last many hours or days. Similar trouble may follow the dangerous procedure of 'manipulation' of an arthritic cervical spine, which is practised by osteopaths, and, regrettably, by some medically qualified practitioners.

Other Causes of Vertigo

Tumours of the brain stem and IVth ventricle, especially in childhood, disturb the vestibular nuclei and cause vertigo. An acute relapse of disseminated sclerosis affecting the brain stem may cause severe vertigo and vomiting lasting several days. Very occasionally vertigo may occur as part of an attack of temporal lobe epilepsy, and attacks similar to vertigo can be a symptom of a psychoneurosis.

DISTURBANCES OF SLEEP

How normal sleep and waking occur is not quite certain. As lesions of the reticular formation (p. 45) can produce a state resembling sleep, it is likely that sleep is brought about when this formation stops sending alerting impulses to the cerebral cortex.

Insomnia is rarely a sign of organic nervous disease, and commonly a sign of psychoneurosis. Some degree is normal in old age, and it occurs in many feverish and toxic states. In certain types of encephalitis, especially encephalitis lethargica, sleep rhythm is reversed, the patients being drowsy during the day and very wakeful and troublesome during the night. Increased sleepiness, or **hypersomnia,** is common in fatigue, and while taking sedative drugs, and may become very severe when there is a rise in intracranial pressure due to cerebral tumour, or brain swelling.

Narcolepsy is a condition usually affecting rather plump adults in which they are suddenly overcome by **irresistible sleepiness,** often under embarrassing circumstances. They may fall asleep in the middle of a meal, and under monotonous circumstances such as while driving. A touch will arouse them and they do not feel sleepy in between times. Narcoleptics also suffer from four other conditions. (1) **Sleep paralysis;** here the 'mind' wakes up before the body, and for some minutes after waking the patient is unable to move his limbs. This occurs sometimes in normal people. (2) **Dream hallucinations** in which the patient wakes, but a dream seems to continue, so that they think people or animals are in the bedroom. (3) **Somnambulism** (sleep walking) when the body wakes up before the mind. (4) **Cataplexy;** this is a condition in which, on intense emotion, such as fright, a burst of **laughter** or of crying, the patient's knees give way and he falls helpless to the ground. 'I laughed till I dropped.' This must not be confused with catalepsy, which is a psychogenic trance-like state, often affecting young females, lasting hours or days, and very rarely seen nowadays.

Treatment

Narcolepsy remains perhaps the only condition for which it is justified to prescribe regular dosage of **amphetamine,** usually as dextro-amphetamine, but cataplexy is greatly helped by imipramine and narcolepsy itself may be improved.

16 *EPILEPSY*

Nerve cells function by discharging small electrical waves. Those discharges arising from the brain can be measured by the **electroencephalograph,** or E.E.G., which is described further in Chap. 20. If the brain cells suddenly produce a burst of very much larger electrical waves than normal, then an epileptic fit may result. Patients whose brains have a tendency to do this repeatedly are said to suffer from epilepsy. This tendency is sometimes weakly hereditary; or it may develop from an area of damaged issue. These two main types of epilepsy are called **'idiopathic'** and **'symptomatic'.**

Idiopathic Epilepsy

As the name suggests, the exact cause for the electrical abnormality in this group is unknown. Microscopic examination of the brain at post-mortem shows no abnormality, but there may be some biochemical abnormality in the cells. The tendency seems to be passed on through certain families for many generations, some members developing fits, but most having none. The fits start in **childhood, adolescence** (especially around puberty), or early adult life; they take the form of either **generalised convulsions,** or **petit mal attacks** (these terms are explained below) and the patient is usually normal in between attacks. There is often a **family history.**

Symptomatic Epilepsy

Here the fits are one of the symptoms of **brain damage** or **disease.** As methods of neurological investigation have improved, more and more cases once considered 'idiopathic' have been transferred into this group. The suspicion that epileptic attacks are symptomatic arises when (a) the attacks start **later** in life (over the age of 30); (b) they are **focal** (see below); (c) there are **abnormal signs** in between attacks, or shortly after an attack. These patients do not have true petit mal, and there is no family history. Other symptoms of the brain disease may, of course, also be present, and any of the diseases affecting the brain already described may be the cause. One is particularly on the alert for the possibility of a **tumour,** for removal may cure the patient.

TYPES OF EPILEPTIC FIT

In either of the two main types of epilepsy described above, several different types of fit may occur.

Grand Mal Attacks

A grand mal, or major, fit may start abruptly with loss of consciousness, or there may be a short warning or **aura.** The type of aura is important, for it shows where in the brain the abnormal discharge starts. In a generalised fit there is often a vague indescribable sensation, followed by loss of consciousness, and **rigid** contraction of all muscles. The arms are flexed, the legs extended, the head thrown back or turned to one side, the teeth tightly clenched, so that the **tongue** or cheek may be **bitten,** and respiratory movements checked, so that the patient becomes **cyanosed.** This is called the **tonic** phase. After a few moments, the **clonic** phase begins. The muscles of the face, limbs and trunk develop a coarse jerking, which may become violent. There is often **incontinence** of urine and occasionally of faeces. Breathing then becomes **stertorous,** the face flushes, the muscles relax, but the patient remains deeply unconscious, unrousable, with absent corneal and pupillary reflexes, and extensor plantars. This **post-epileptic coma** may last from ten minutes to several hours. It is followed by a period of confusion, and often by deep but apparently normal, **sleep.** During the period of confusion the patient may be restless, and may wander around doing things automatically (**post-epileptic automatism**), but, knowing nothing of it, may be a danger to himself or to others.

By no means all grand mal attacks show all the features described above. There may merely be sudden loss of consciousness; or loss of consciousness with rigidity, but no clonic movements; or almost any combination of the symptoms mentioned. They may be so mild as to consist only of incontinence of urine at night, or so severe that the patient suffocates and dies.

Generalised attacks may be idiopathic or symptomatic.

Jacksonian Attacks

Hughlings Jackson described fits starting by twitching of the mouth, thumb, or big toe, and spreading to other areas of the same side, then passing over to the other side, and ending in loss of consciousness. These attacks are **symptomatic** of **irritation** of the **cerebral cortex** by a tumour, scar tissue, or some form of inflammation.

Focal Epileptic Attacks

Focal attacks affect just one part of the body, Jacksonian attacks are a form of focal epilepsy, but many focal attacks show no spread, never become generalised, nor cause loss of consciousness. They are always **symptomatic** of a **localised cerebral lesion** and the form the attack takes depends on where the lesion lies. It is therefore, vital to have an accurate account of the fits. A lesion in the motor cortex will cause convulsive twitching of parts of the opposite side of the body, and this is often followed by a temporary paralysis of the parts involved **(Todd's paralysis).** In the sensory cortex it will cause tingling or numbness of arm, leg, or face; in the occipital lobe, flashes of light in the opposite visual field; in the temporal lobe, vivid scenes, curious sensations of smell or of taste, and often a feeling that this is all very familiar—the so-called **déjà-vu phenomenon.** These may be the only symptoms of the fit, or they may be followed by unconsciousness and a generalised fit.

Psychomotor Epilepsy

The abnormal discharge may sometimes merely cause a sudden **disturbance of behaviour.** The patient may start running round in a circle, or fighting someone, or vigorously rearranging objects. This will stop equally suddenly, and there is no knowledge of what has happened. Attacks of this type originate in the temporal lobes, and may be preceded by the hallucinations of taste, smell or vision mentioned above. They are, of course, possibly dangerous, but in fact rarely are.

Petit Mal Attacks

The term **'petit mal'** is often loosely used in practice to describe short-lived epileptic attacks of any type. This is quite wrong. They are a very special type of attack, always **idiopathic** and require a special form of treatment.

They start in childhood and adolescence, only occasionally persisting into adult life. **Many** attacks occur each day, sometimes hundreds. Each consists of a momentary loss of touch with the surroundings (the French use the word **'absence'**) so that the child pauses in conversation, the eyelids may flicker, the head nod, something may be dropped, words or figures may be repeated, and then the child picks up the conversation and only a close observer realises that anything has been wrong. Such attacks show a **characteristic E.E.G.** abnormality (see p. 178), and their treatment is quite different from that of grand mal epilepsy.

Myoclonic Attacks

Myoclonus is a **shock-like jerking** of the muscles. This may happen in the arms in many epileptics, especially first thing in the morning, and it sometimes occurs without other signs of epilepsy. Similar jerks just on dropping off to sleep occur in normal people. Repeated myoclonus is seen in several diffuse diseases of the brain, including subacute encephalitis.

Hypsarrhythmia

This name is given to a gross E.E.G. abnormality seen in infants subject to fits, especially the so-called **'salaam' seizures** in which the child throws the arms back and then repeatedly bends head and body forwards.

Post-traumatic Epilepsy

Epilepsy may follow serious injury to the brain, and all types of attack, except petit mal, may be seen. Fits immediately after the injury, due to cerebral bruising, are not of much importance, but when they develop later, usually within the first two years, they are due to **cerebral scarring** and may recur for many years. They are most common if an injury has penetrated the dura and brain, and are very rare if there was no unconsciousness and no fracture.

Status Epilepticus

Epileptic attacks usually occur at well spaced intervals, but sometimes one fit passes into the next so quickly that **consciousness** is **not regained** and the attacks may last for **many hours.** The **temperature** rises to hyperpyrexial levels, and unless vigorously treated (p. 142) the patient may become exhausted and die. Though more common in idiopathic epilepsy, it may occasionally occur as a result of structural disease and if an adult never having had epilepsy, suddenly goes into status epilepticus this often indicates a cerebral tumour. The epileptic may develop status epilepticus during some **intercurrent illness,** but it is a particular danger if treatment is suddenly **discontinued.**

THE INVESTIGATION OF EPILEPSY

First an accurate and detailed **history** must be obtained from the patient and the relatives. Secondly a full examination is carried out. If a **fit** occurs while under observation it must be carefully **recorded,** and the part the nurse can play in this is described on p. 187. An **electroencephalogram** will be carried out in most cases. This may show, in between attacks, the type of abnormality which from experience is known to be present in epileptics; it may show a clear cut petit mal attack; it may show that abnormal discharges arise from one point only, therefore suggesting a lesion of the brain at that point and requiring further investigation still.

In-patient investigation should be carried out on all cases in which (a) the attacks are **focal,** or Jacksonian, or arise from the temporal lobe; (b) the aura suggests a single **focal** origin; (c) there is a post-epileptic **paralysis**; (d) there are **abnormal signs** between attacks; (e) the **E.E.G.** shows a localised abnormality. The most helpful investigations are C.A.T. scanning, arteriography, radioisotope brain scanning and air-encephalography which shows tumours, angiomas, or atrophy, and possibly special E.E.G. techniques (p. 178) in the temporal lobe attacks. Such full studies are not necessarily indicated if abnormalities are known to have been present since birth or an old head injury.

THE TREATMENT OF A FIT

Once a fit has started nothing will work quickly enough to stop it, and the immediate treatment is to **prevent** the patient **injuring** himself and to ensure that his breathing is not obstructed. A firm object is placed between the teeth as soon as a fit begins, and the patient should be moved away from fire, water, traffic, heights, walls, or articles of furniture on which he might injure himself during the convulsion. The clothing should be loosened, the collar undone, the tongue must not fall into the back of the throat, nor the head into a cushion or pillow to cause suffocation. On recovery the patient must not be left alone in case post-epileptic automatism develops.

Prevention of Further Fits

Symptomatic epilepsy has a demonstrable cause and attempts have to be made to **eliminate** this **cause,** e.g. removal of a benign tumour. If it is not possible to correct the underlying condition, e.g. in cerebral atrophy, then the treatment is the same in the symptomatic and idiopathic types.

For grand mal, **phenobarbitone** forms the basis of treatment. This is often combined with **Epanutin** (phenytain), being in practice if not in theory, a more effective combination. **Primidone** (mysoline) is another effective drug and there are many more for which great claim is made. Most of these are no better than those already mentioned, but in cases of temporal lobe attacks **carbamazepine** (Tegretol), mainly used for trigeminal neuralgia, may sometimes be gratifyingly beneficial. More recently the preparation **sodium valproate** (Epilim) is being used in patients failing to respond to other measures. The results are sometimes dramatic, but its combination with other drugs very easily produces toxic effects. **Sulthiame** (Ospolot) is another drug particularly inclined to produce toxic symptoms when combined with epanutin or mysoline.

These drugs, with the exception of Epilim, do not influence petit mal. Here **Epilim** and the **suximides** are the preparations of choice. Epilim is perhaps one of the most effective but toxicity is a problem and the suximides are preferred by many, **ethosuximide** being most commonly used. The **-diones** introduced earlier are still required in some patients (tridione, paradione) but have more toxic effects. As many children starting with petit mal may develop grand mal later it is always wise to combine ethosuximide treatment with preventative doses of phenobarbitone.

The usual dosage of these various drugs is given below:

Barbiturates

Phenobarbitone 30–60 mg b.d. or t.d.s.
Phenobarbitone as spansules 100 mg daily or b.d.

Hydantoins

Phenytoin sodium (Epanutin) 100 mg b.d. or t.d.s.

Primidone (Mysoline) 250 mg t.d.s.
Carbamazepine (Tegretol) 100–200 mg t.d.s.

-diones

Trimethadione (Tridione) 0·3 g t.d.s. or more
Paramethadione (Paradione) 0·3 g t.d.s. or more

Suximides

Ethosuximide (Zarontin) 250 mg t.d.s. or more
Phenosuximide (Milontin) 250 mg t.d.s. or more
Sodium Valproate (Epilim) 200–400 mg t.d.s.

Absolute regularity and adequate dosage are essential. Estimating of the blood levels of the drugs will indicate whether dosage is adequate, too low, or indeed too high. No reduction of treatment should be made until there has been complete freedom from fits for an absolute minimum of **two years,** however long this may take. **Suddenly stopping treatment often precipitates status epilepticus, which can be fatal.**

Treatment of Status Epilepticus

The greatest danger in status epilepticus comes from inadequate breathing resulting in **lack of oxygen** for brain cells and permanent damage. Ensuring a **free airway** is first priority. Protection of the patient from injury is vital as is prevention or treatment of the **hyperpyrexia** which is common. This can be done by tepid sponging, spirit spraying or nursing under a moistened sheet on which a fan blows a constant current of air. The patient should not be left alone for a moment during status.

Diazepam (Valium) given **intravenously** at the rate, for adults, of 1 mgm per minute is the treatment of choice. After 10 mgm the fits are often brought under control and time allowed for setting up an intravenous drip into which further diazepam, or intravenous barbiturates or hydantoins can be given. The dangers of this treatment are the production of very low blood pressure and the exaggeration of the effects of any other drugs that the patient may already be taking.

Paraldehyde given **intramuscularly** in doses of 10 ml repeated in half an hour is another very effective measure and this can be given in 10% solution into a saline drip.

Often the patient will go into prolonged and deep unconsciousness after a period of status, partly as a result of cumulative medication, and all the measures required for nursing an unconscious patient apply, even to the extent of intubation and the use of antibiotics to prevent chest infection.

In some patients who completely fail to respond the use of **curare** to paralyse the patient completely, combined with **controlled artificial respiration,** may be required, provided a trained team is available and constantly present.

Gradually intravenous dosage will be replaced by oral medication with the usual anticonvulsants and the patient be allowed gradually to regain consciousness.

Toxic Effects of Anti-epileptic Drugs

Barbiturates and Mysoline cause drowsiness, which is overcome by persisting with the treatment. Mysoline sometimes causes abdominal pain, vomiting and dilated pupils. Large doses of Epanutin cause hypertrophy of the gums. Tegretol and the -diones occasionally cause disturbances of blood cell formation, sometimes even **agranulocytosis.** Combinations of drugs tend to interact with each other. Phenobarbitone and Epanutin in too heavy dosage cause **ataxia, nystagmus, dysarthria,** confusion and a mental euphoria which resembles drunkenness. Sulthiame is particularly inclined to increase the side effects of Epanutin. Combination of these drugs can disturb **folic acid** metabolism and produce **macrocytic anaemia** which can be corrected by giving folic acid. There has been some evidence that Epanutin taken during pregnancy may rarely be associated with congenital deformities in infants, but this is of such rarity that adequate control of fits during pregnancy is of much greater importance. Fear of these rare effects must never prevent adequate dosage, which is the dosage which effectively prevents fits. Providing it is not producing toxic effects the actual amount is not so important.

Surgery in the Treatment of Epilepsy

If the epilepsy is caused by accessible tumours, vascular malformations or other benign conditions, their removal is obviously indicated, though drug control of epilepsy may still be required for years post-operatively. Some extensive angiomas in infants (e.g. **the Sturge-Weber syndrome** may be treated by hemispherectomy, i.e. the removal of the major portion of one cerebral hemisphere, the other hemisphere apparently being capable of taking over the role of both if dealt with early enough in life.

Surgery may also be employed (a) to **excise** ragged **scar** tissue in post-traumatic epilepsy; and (b) in cases of **temporal lobe epilepsy,** when removing part of the temporal lobe may stop fits completely. Before considering surgery, however, it must be certain that the fits arise from a single focus; that they are so frequent that they are completely disrupting the patient's life; and that adequate treatment has completely failed.

Prognosis

Epileptic fits usually diminish with age, and often cease altogether in middle life. Unfortunately, a few patients are completely uncontrollable, deteriorate steadily, and may have to be cared for in an institution. Petit mal very rarely troubles patients in adult life.

Advice to Epileptics

There are many problems which worry the epileptic and the wisest answers to their queries are given in Chap. 22, p. 189.

Nothing is worse for young patients than the feeling that people are constantly 'looking after' them, waiting for the next attack, always protecting them and encouraging the suspicion they have themselves that there is something different about them, something that is perhaps rather disgraceful. Remember that anybody's brain can, under certain circumstances, produce the electrical discharge which causes a fit—the only difference is that an epileptic brain will do this frequently by itself, unless suppressed by appropriate treatment. There is no more disgrace in being an epileptic than in having migraine, and that is a highly respectable disorder.

17 *DISEASES OF MUSCLE*

The muscles are a vital part of the motor system, and diseases affecting them have always come within the province of the neurologist, even if the nervous system is normal. It is, in fact, not always easy to tell whether muscle weakness and wasting is due to a lesion of the motor nerves or to disease limited to the muscle itself. Muscle diseases may be degenerative, when they are called **myopathies,** or more commonly nowadays, **muscular dystrophies**; or they may be inflammatory—**myositis.** In addition, there is a remarkable condition called **myasthenia gravis,** in which impulses cannot 'get across' from the nerve into the muscle it supplies.

THE MUSCULAR DYSTROPHIES OR MYOPATHIES

The myopathies are **heredo-familial** diseases in which the muscle fibres slowly degenerate and **waste,** eventually producing grave disability. As they are often replaced by **fat,** the patient superficially may not look very wasted. There are several different types, varying in the age groups and particular muscles affected, and in the gravity of the prognosis.

Pseudohypertrophic Muscular Dystrophy

Also known as the **Duchenne** type, this is the most serious form of muscular dystrophy. It is almost, though not entirely, confined to boys, and progression is such that very few reach adult life. It is given this name because though they are weak, the muscles look **unusually large,** or hypertrophied, and some of the fibres actually become larger than normal before they become wasted, while others are replaced by an excess of fat.

Mode of Inheritance. Though mainly affecting boys the disease is passed on by apparently unaffected females, i.e. by relatives who 'carry' the disease. Most of these female carriers can now be detected by the combination of chemical, electrical and biopsy examination of their muscles, and advice has to be given regarding the dangers of transmission, because there is an almost 50% chance of any son of a female carrier being affected, and a high chance of a daughter being herself a carrier.

Symptoms

The parents first notice that the child walks badly, and has difficulty in picking himself up after falling, and in climbing stairs. They often express surprise at their son's increasing disability 'when his muscles seem so well developed'.

Signs

The child walks with a **waddle** and has marked **lordosis.** The calves, buttocks and shoulder girdle **muscles** look much **larger** than expected for his age, and have a tough rubbery feel, but may,

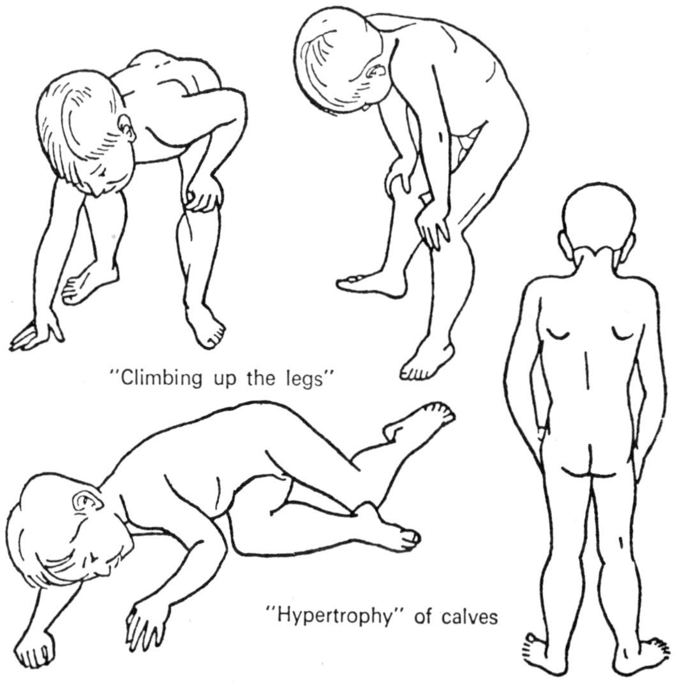

FIG. 17.1 A child with pseudohypertrophic muscular dystrophy, showing the method of standing upright.

in fact, be very weak. The back muscles are weak, and if the child is told to stand up after lying on the floor, he will do it in a very characteristic manner (Fig. 17.1). First rolling on to his face, he will then half kneel, place his hands first on his ankles, and then on his shins, his knees, his thighs and so gradually push himself upright. This is called **'climbing up the legs'.** The tendon reflexes are usually absent. The facial muscles are rarely affected. Gradually the pseudohypertrophy gives way to wasting and the patients die eventually of chest infection.

Diagnosis

The blood level of a muscle enzyme called **creatine phosphokinase** (C.P.K.) is considerably raised, in the disease, and also in an apparently unaffected boy who later will develop the disease. This may also be slightly raised in carriers. Electromyography (p. 178) shows typical myopathic features. Muscle biopsy shows enlargement of some muscle fibres, wasting of others and replacement by fat.

Facio-Scapulo-Humeral Dystrophy

As the name suggests, the wasting and weakness affects the **face, shoulder girdles** and **upper arms,** often on one side more than the other. It develops in adult life, is the **least grave** of the dystrophies, progresses slowly, and is compatible with quite long life. The muscles do not hypertrophy. It is inherited from an affected individual, not through carriers.

Limb-Girdle Dystrophy

Again affecting older patients, the muscles involved are those of the **hip girdle,** the **shoulder girdle,** or both. Weakness and wasting progresses slowly, and disability is considerable within ten years. There is usually no history in preceding generations.

Ocular Myopathy

In late middle life (and very occasionally earlier) degenerative changes may develop in the **lids** and **eye muscles.** This results in progressive ptosis and difficulty in moving the eyes, until they finally become **fixed** in the midline. It used to be thought that this was due to degeneration of the nuclei in the midbrain, and was called progressive nuclear ophthalmoplegia, but the lesion is now known to lie in the muscles. There is no treatment, though a plastic operation may be needed to raise the lids.

Treatment of the Myopathies

No curative treatment is known. Physiotherapy is usually of little use and may overtire the weakened muscles. Supports may be needed for the back, but they must be light enough for the weak muscles to carry them. The patients are very prone to chest infections, which may prove fatal, so that care is needed during even a common cold.

The **Muscular Dystrophy Association** has branches in all regions, and spend large sums of money on research into these terrible diseases. They also can help patients to obtain chairs and household appliances which make their lot a little easier.

MYOTONIA

Myotonia is the name given to a condition in which muscles continue to contract for some time after the need for that contraction has passed. It is most strikingly seen in the two diseases—dystrophia myotonica and myotonia congenita.

Dystrophia Myotonica (myotonia atrophica)

This is a heredo-familial disorder which affects men more than women, and appears to start in adult life.

Symptoms

The patients usually complain of increasing **weakness** of the hands and arms, and occasionally of muscular **wasting.** Very occasionally they have noticed **difficulty in 'letting-go'** after picking something up, or when shaking hands. They rarely complain of the many features which are found on examination, but may realise that their vision is failing.

Signs

The appearance is very characteristic, and all patients look alike. They have long thin faces, with **drooping** of the **eyelids** and the corners of the mouth. They go **bald** early and their remaining hair is unkempt. The **sternomastoids** are wasted, giving the neck a scraggy appearance, and they can only raise their heads with difficulty from the pillow. Most muscles show some wasting, but especially the hand and thigh muscles. The **myotonia** is shown when the patient smiles, for the smile will remain after the face should have relaxed. If he grips something he is unable to loosen the grip afterwards, and has to drag his hand away. Tapping the tongue, or some other muscle, causes a dent which remains for an appreciable time. There are a number of other abnormalities such as **cataracts,** atrophy of the **testes,** and sometimes **cardiac defects.**

Treatment

Nothing halts the steady progression of weakness and wasting, but the course varies greatly. In some patients myotonia is a greater problem than weakness and if relieved the patient is helped considerably. **Quinine** was originally used, but regular dosage of **procaine amide** is more effective, and an injection of a long-acting preparation of **A.C.T.H.** will reduce the myotonia within 4 hours, though the effect lasts only for 24 hours to 3 days.

Myotonia Congenita

This is also a hereditary condition, but the myotonia is present from **infancy,** and dystrophic features, i.e. muscle wasting, baldness, cataracts, atrophy of testes or ovaries, are usually absent. The myotonia may improve as the patient gets older. These patients complain more of the muscular stiffness than of weakness, and are, therefore, even more helped if the myotonia can be relieved.

OTHER MUSCLE DISORDERS

Myositis

Muscles can become infected from dirty wounds, or careless injections, by parasites, or by infected emboli. They will then become swollen and tender as inflammatory cells pour into them from the blood. The myositis described here is not, however, due to infection. Whether it is an allergic or a toxic state is not certain, but it can occur with similar inflammatory lesions of the skin (**dermatomyositis**), or of the blood vessels (**polyarteritis nodosa**). When many muscles are involved we speak of **polymyositis.**

Symptoms

The patients, of any age, feel generally unwell and complain of increasing **weakness** of the limbs with **swelling** and **tenderness** of the muscles.

Signs

There is slight fever and a raised pulse rate. The affected muscles are weak and very tender, and the overlying skin may be a little swollen. The tendon reflexes are absent. The blood sedimentation rate is high and the serum level of the enzymes aldolase and creatine kinase are raised. The muscles may waste if the disease has been present for a long time. The diagnosis is usually confirmed by **biopsy** of one of the affected muscles, when oedema and infiltration with inflammatory cells will be seen.

Treatment

A.C.T.H. and steroids, often requiring high dosage, can cause considerable improvement, but treatment is prolonged and the prognosis not always good. Some patients with polymyositis are harbouring a previously unsuspected carcinoma.

Myasthenia Gravis

Myasthenia means weakness of muscles, but the term is usually used for a **weakness** which rapidly **worsens** as the muscle is used, and rapidly recovers when the muscle is at rest. Myasthenia gravis mainly affects young women, but can occur in either sex at any age. It is caused by an abnormality preventing impulses passing across the point where the finest branches of the motor nerves end in the muscle fibres—**the neuromuscular junction.**

Symptoms

The eyes are often first affected. The **eyelids** droop, the eyes squint, and there is **double vision.** These all **vary** from hour to hour. The patients may be normal on first waking, but get worse as the day goes on. The voice becomes weak and **hoarse** towards the end of each sentence; **chewing** and **swallowing** become increasingly difficult as a meal progresses. The arm and back muscles become weak after use, vary enormously, recover completely on resting, at times appearing quite normal. Sometimes many months may pass with no symptoms of any sort.

Signs

Any muscle may be affected, so that the signs vary greatly. Ptosis, squinting, hoarseness and a nasal voice are the most common, all these features varying from minute to minute during the examination. The essential sign is the ease with which muscles become **fatigued.** If a patient looks upwards without blinking for several minutes, the lids gradually droop and may close completely. Fatigue of the voice can be shown by listening to it fading away while the patient reads; and of the arms by making the patient raise them 20–30 times. A short period of rest is then given when the power may become normal in what a few moments before had been an almost paralysed muscle.

The diagnosis can be confirmed by giving a subcutaneous injection of **neostigmine (prostigmine)** (2·5 mg) together with 0·6 mg atropine. The weak muscles become nearly normal within 45 minutes, and this improvement lasts 4–5 hours. The **edrophonium**

chloride (Tensilon) test is quicker; 1 ml (10 mg) given intravenously, restores power to normal in one minute, but the effect usually lasts for less than 5 minutes, though sometimes much longer.

Treatment

Prostigmine, or the longer-acting **pyridostigmine,** must be taken regularly by mouth. To keep the patient well the dose may have to be very large and taken very frequently. Most patients respond well, though improvement in the eye muscles is sometimes disappointing. The dose may have to be raised during colds, chest infections, etc., for the patient may find difficulty in coughing. In some cases, however, nothing seems to halt the advance of the disease, and paralysis of throat and respiratory muscles develops. The patient then will need the prostigmine by injection every one or two hours; will probably have to have a tracheotomy, and perhaps even artificial respiration. Even from this precarious state improvement is always possible.

Removal of the **thymus** gland helps some patients, especially young women, if medical treatment seems to be failing, but the results can never be predicted with certainty. If a tumour of the thymus is present the outlook is very bad.

A.C.T.H. may also improve some of the more severe cases, which might be taken as support of the theory that myasthenia gravis falls into the ever widening group of so-called 'auto-immune' diseases.

18 *PRINCIPLES OF OPERATIVE NEURO-SURGERY*

The central nervous system differs from other parts of the body in many respects, and these differences affect the technique and nature of the operative surgery of the central nervous system. The first special feature is obviously the need to approach the brain and spinal cord by opening the skull, or through a laminectomy of the spinal vertebrae. The presence of a rigid container around the brain and spinal cord is one of the reasons that **pressure** is so easily transmitted to these structures by any additional **space-occupying lesion** within the bony casing. This may be a **tumour, abscess, haemorrhage,** or a **swollen** brain or spinal cord, due to **inflammation, oedema,** or a combination of these, as in brain injury. It is therefore a prime concern of the neurosurgeon to avoid pressure occurring within the skull, and to a lesser extent in the spine at any time. Small amounts of haemorrhage or oedema, which could be tolerated in almost any other part of the body, may be fatal.

The brain and spinal cord are extremely sensitive to **deprivation of oxygen,** whether this is of remote origin, as might be the case with a lung lesion, imperfect anaesthesia or blood loss, or of local origin from arterial occlusion or pressure on the brain or cord. It is well known that total deprivation of oxygen will cause irreparable brain damage *within four minutes,* but it is sometimes forgotten that very slight degrees of oxygen lack also have their effect on the function of nerve cells. For instance, a retractor held against the brain for an hour or two may irrevocably damage the cells that lie beneath it, unless it is relaxed from time to time in order to allow circulation through the underlying capillaries. This reminds one of the particular sensitivity of the nervous system to **damage by instruments.** The brain should never be retracted except with a flat instrument protected by cottonoid, and the same applies even more to the spinal cord, which should not be touched at all unless this is unavoidable. Nerves should only be held with hooks or retractors, and never picked up with forceps. They may be retracted with broad tape, and occasionally the larger ones may be handled with fine forceps applied only to the fibrous covering of the nerves.

Throughout the book, attention has been drawn to the effects of raised intracranial tension on the central brain structures where they pass through the opening in the tentorium (the shelf of the dura mater separating the cerebral hemispheres from the cerebellum), and at the foramen magnum at the base of the skull. When operating, it is extremely important not to open the thick dural lining membrane (dura mater) surrounding the brain unless the pressure within is normal, or has been reduced to a suitable level. If it is opened while the pressure within is still high, the brain will extrude like toothpaste, causing serious damage. Temporary lowering of pressure can often be brought about by removing cerebro-spinal fluid from a cerebral ventricle, or by removing water from the brain tissues by **osmotherapy** (see p. 180). Alteration of the blood gases by **controlled respiration,** and the position of the patient's head are also important. During controlled respiration the patient's natural breathing is paralysed but it is carried on through an **endotracheal tube** connected to **a mechanical respirator.** The anaesthetist can control the rate at which the patient breathes, the depth of each breath, and the pressure and nature of the gases which are given. This makes a considerable difference to the tension of the brain, which can also be slightly lowered by raising the head. The brain should never be lower than the heart when it is being operated upon, in order to aid the return of venous blood and to prevent congestion.

These general principles are further governed by the nature of cerebral and spinal **blood-vessels.** Although there is a small but very inefficient amount of anastomosis between the end arteries of the brain, this only comes into effect when occlusion is gradual. The **Circle of Willis** at the base of the brain continually forms an efficient main artery **anastomosis** in most people. However, it does not always do so, either because of congenital variations in the arteries or as a result of spasm. With these exceptions, occlusion of a cerebral artery will usually cause the death of cells in the territory it supplies. Anastomosis between spinal cord arteries is more effective than between cerebral vessels; though this depends on the level, for some areas of the cord are dependent on single arteries for their survival. **The surface vessels** of the central nervous system are extremely **delicate** and will tear, even with the gentlest handling. Furthermore, they are often not supported by surrounding tissues as they are in many other parts of the body. The result is that any arterial bleeding spreads quite rapidly in the subarachnoid or subdural spaces, or even in the soft brain tissues. The delicate nature of even the **arterial vessels** makes it impossible to grasp them with artery forceps in order to apply a ligature, and they have to be occluded by **coagulation with diathermy** or by the application of little metal **clips** that grip them and are left in place on the cut end (Fig. 18.1). **Venous bleeding** is also controlled by diathermy, but if the vessels are small it may be possible to stop haemorrhage by the application of **gelatine foam,** or a stamp of **beaten muscle.**

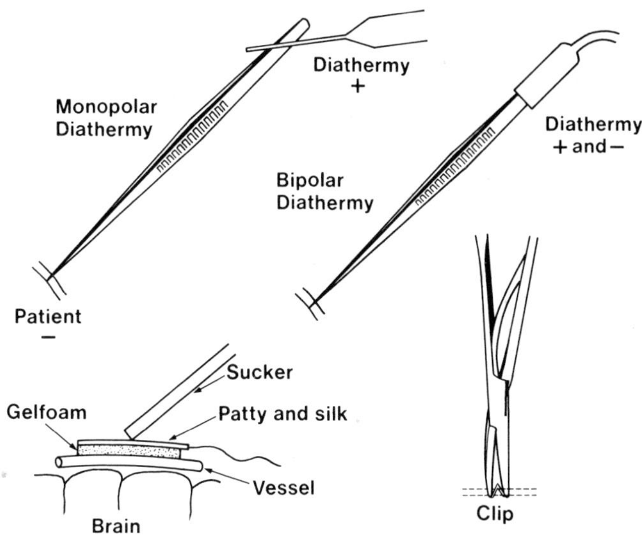

FIG. 18.1 Methods of stopping bleeding from cerebral arteries and veins.

In the case of bleeding from a dural venous sinus, either of the last two methods are generally used or it may be possible to close an opening in the sinus by clips or sutures. During the control of haemorrhage, suction is essential in order to be able to see the bleeding point. **Suction** is usually applied with a fine metal or glass sucker through a cottonoid pledget (**patty**) which may have a perforated plastic film on one side to prevent it adhering to the clot or brain, this also stops the brain being drawn into the sucker (Fig. 18.1).

The tissues of the central nervous system are very susceptible to **drying,** being normally bathed in cerebro-spinal fluid. The heat from an operating lamp is often quite significant, and this increases the normal evaporation from exposed tissues. It is therefore necessary to irrigate the brain frequently during an operation with isotonic fluid at body temperature. The absolute necessity for the fluid to be completely sterile cannot be over-emphasised. **Ringer's solution** is generally employed.

Infection is another serious problem for the neurosurgeon. Unlike many parts of the body, bacteria do not normally inhabit the nervous system, which cannot tolerate even a mild infection. The central nervous system is less adapted to the control of infection than elsewhere, although it has a special arrangement for doing it. Infection tends to spread rapidly, aided by the cerebro-spinal fluid circulation. This causes **meningitis** and **encephalitis.** When there is localised infection in the brain, an **abscess** can form. This not only occupies space because of its own bulk, but also because of the surrounding oedema. The artificial shunts (see p. 164) used to transport cerebro-spinal fluid away from enlarged ventricles (e.g. hydrocephalus) are made of plastic and silicone rubber, and they form a perfect hide-out for organisms to breed in, where culture conditions are ideal and they are safe from any defence mechanism. The **absolute sterility** of valves and tubing is essential.

We have been considering the special features of the nervous system which make neurosurgical operations different from those on other parts of the body. The effects of this kind of surgery also have peculiarities of their own. Because of the distribution of nerve fibres to and from the spinal cord and brain to every other part of the body, damage to a **very small area** of the brain or cord can produce a **wide area of disability.** Similarly, a very small lesion can cause loss of the power of speech (aphasia) or inability to calculate or perform skilled tasks. It is therefore very important to know which hemisphere is dominant (responsible for speech) and where certain functions are localised. This cannot always be discovered by looking at the brain, and electrical stimulation (among other things) may be necessary in order to find out. In this way, one endeavours to limit the amount of damage that may have to be inflicted in order to remove a tumour etc. to areas which are least likely to cause symptoms. The same principles have to be considered before occluding any blood vessel. *Because of this, one often has to weigh the risks of operation and its after effects, against the risks of a more conservative approach.*

Injury to the **cerebral cortex** and deep tissues can cause **epilepsy,** and this may be the result of **operative damage** as well as being a possible effect of damage caused by a **scar, tumour, haemorrhage** or **injury.** Even at a remote period of time, epilepsy may result from cortical tears and adhesions to the meninges. One can only reduce the risks to the minimum by careful technique, clean incisions, neat scars, and the repair of **dural gaps or defects. Skull defects** should be repaired if they are more than about 1·5 cm in diameter. In the case of larger openings this is necessary to support the brain and prevent undue movement quite apart from cosmetic considerations. Missing bone can be replaced by **acrylic resin, metal plates** (tantalum) or **bone grafts.** Dural defects are repaired with fascia lata, temporalis fascia, pericranium, or preserved (freeze-dried) dura. Brain must never be in direct contact with the scalp without any intervening tissues or substitutes. If this is allowed to happen, there is a risk of damage to the brain which tends to protrude, and if the wound breaks down it leaks cerebro-spinal fluid and forms a brain hernia or fungus. This is often fatal and always difficult to treat. Epilepsy is usually a sequel too.

One has to remember that the **air sinuses** in the skull are a potential source of infection, that they are effectively 'external', and so any fracture involving them falls into the 'compound' category. It is therefore necessary to occlude any opening into an air cell or sinus during an operation, which is done by a free fascial graft or a dural flap. This also prevents leakage of cerebro-spinal fluid through the nose (**rhinorrhoea**). Fractures involving these cavities often have brain or meninges trapped in them, providing a route along which infection can travel inwards, to produce meningitis or a brain abscess.

Finally, we have to remember that brain damage may cause **metabolic disturbances** in the body as a whole. The pituitary gland and stalk, and the overlying hypothalamus are obviously the commonest sources of this kind of problem, even when they are not the target for surgical attack.

When tumours in the **posterior fossa** (whether in the fourth ventricle, cerebellum, or arising from nerves or brain stem) are manipulated during operations for their removal, disturbance of **medullary** function may be caused. These effects are similar to those produced by raised intracranial pressure causing '**coning**' (see pp. 46 and 171). The pulse and respiration are slowed and the blood pressure is raised on account of interference with the function of the cardiac and respiratory centres in the medulla.

19 *NOTES ON CERTAIN NEUROSURGICAL PROCEDURES*

In this chapter, it is intended only to draw attention to a few important points related to some neurosurgical procedures. For a full description of the operations themselves it is necessary to refer to a textbook of operative surgery.

Anaesthesia

When operating on the brain, it must be as lax as possible in order to gain access to the deeper parts and to reduce the force of any retraction to a minimum. The **tension of brain tissue** during an operation depends very much on the anaesthetist. The advent of **controlled respiration** has improved surgical results and reduced the time required very considerably. As has previously been emphasised, adequate **oxygenation** is vital. Any restriction of the **airway** shows itself at once by an increase in brain size. **Local anaesthesia** is still sometimes used, especially when it is necessary to have the patient's co-operation when localising certain parts of the brain. Apart from the scalp nerves, which are blocked by infiltration with local anaesthetic (such as 2% lignocaine—usually with adrenaline 1:200 000), the only other **pain-sensitive** structures encountered at craniotomy are the **muscles** on which a bone flap may be hinged, and the **arteries** in the **dura mater.** The dura mater itself can be cut painlessly, although **stretching** and **distortion** cause headache. Cutting the bone causes no pain though it may be unpleasantly noisy to the conscious patient. Local anaesthesia is time consuming and a strain for everybody concerned, but it is a way of avoiding the hazards of unreliable anaesthesia in adverse circumstances, and of maintaining communication with the patient during operations.

The Position of the Patient

The standard position for **frontal** and **lateral craniotomy** is with the patient **lying on his back** (**supine**) on the table. If the head has to be turned to one side, it is usually necessary to support the opposite shoulder and hip in order to avoid too much torsion on the rotated neck. Operations on the **postero-lateral** part of the head are often better done with the **patient face down (prone)**, and the head turned to one side. Operations on the **posterior fossa** can be done in this position but the head needs a **special** (e.g. horse-shoe) **head rest** to allow the anaesthetic tubes to pass forwards (Fig. 19.1.).

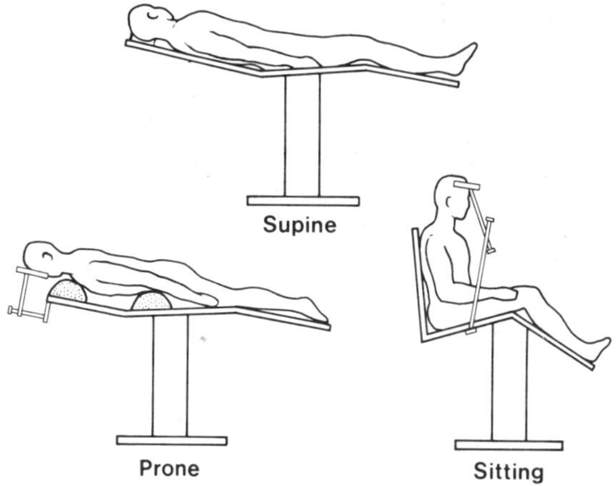

FIG. 19.1 Position of the patient for neurosurgical operations.

Care is needed to avoid pressure on the forehead, eyeballs and cheeks. The pelvis and chest need support in order to allow free abdominal movement. Alternatively, the patient can be fixed in a **sitting position** for access to the **posterior fossa.** The head is then held in a special holder.

When operations are done in this position the pressure in the venous sinuses is often atmospheric or below, so that if a sinus or a venous channel in the bone is opened, it is possible for air to enter the blood stream. The anaesthetist monitors this very dangerous possibility with an oesophageal stethoscope or an ultra-sound apparatus. If it occurs, the patient must be immediately laid flat with the right side of the heart uppermost in order to reduce the likelihood of **air embolism.** The venous pressure should always be raised at intervals when the patient is in the sitting position in order to check the complete control of any bleeding from cut veins. This is done by the anaesthetist. Operations on the **cervical spine** can also be done with the patient sitting, but the hazard of air embolism seems to be a little greater than for craniotomy. The **trigeminal ganglion** is sometimes approached from the temporal region with the patient sitting, but held in a different type of retainer allowing a lateral exposure.

Most neurosurgeons prefer to operate on the spine with the patient prone, as previously described. The head can be turned to one side if the operation site is below the mid-thoracic level. As previously mentioned, the chest and pelvis need to be supported on pillows or special pads in order to allow freedom of movement to the abdominal wall.

When operating on very **small children** it is important to reduce the weight of drapes and instruments around the head as much as possible, or they may tend to squeeze the brain out of a craniotomy wound.

Blood loss at craniotomy is less than it used to be, but it is unwise to operate without **matched blood** in the theatre, for blood loss can be sudden and severe.

Osteoplastic Flaps—Craniotomy

The main principle of **scalp incision** for craniotomy is that a scalp flap providing access to the interior should carry its blood supply through a broad base (Fig. 19.2). The base is therefore usually inferior. **Bone flaps** are made by joining a series of holes in the skull with saw cuts, unless a special side-cutting drill is employed

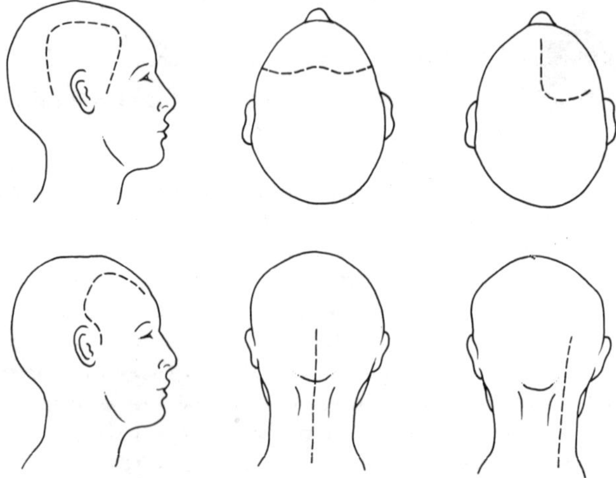

FIG. 19.2 Some incisions commonly used in neurosurgery.

(Fig. 19.3). The bone flaps, being hinged on muscle, turn downwards in the same direction as the scalp flaps. **Dural flaps** are turned in the opposite way with the base adjacent to the nearest venous sinus, usually the sagittal sinus. In the **posterior fossa** a **stellate incision** in the dura mater is sometimes used instead of a flap.

It may sometimes be preferable to remove bone altogether rather than form a bone flap (**craniectomy**). The bone defect need not be repaired if it is under the occipital or temporal muscles. Elsewhere repair may have to be delayed in the case of head injury for fear of

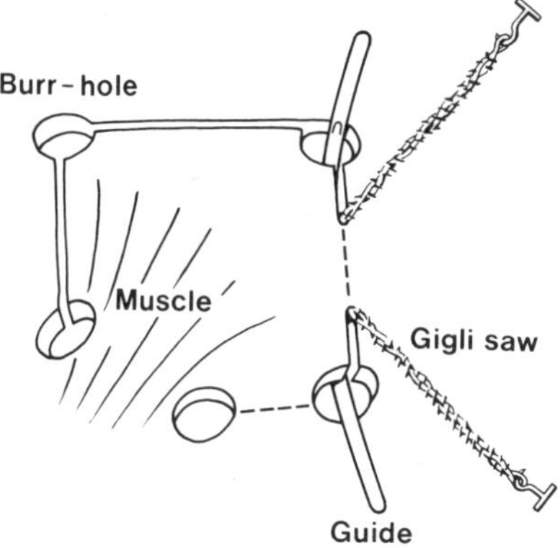

FIG. 19.3 Burr-holes are joined by saw cuts to make an osteoplastic flap.

infection. In many comminuted depressed skull fractures, it is possible to replace the bone fragments after treatment of injuries to the brain and dura.

Burr-holes and Trephine Holes

These are used to penetrate the skull in order to introduce a needle or cannula, for the purpose of removing cerebro-spinal fluid from a ventricle, obtaining a biopsy of a tumour, or removing fluid, pus, or blood. Burr-holes are also the usual means of introducing a wire saw in order to cut a bone flap. The **skull** is first of all penetrated by a **perforator** which makes a conical hole (Fig. 19.4). This is then

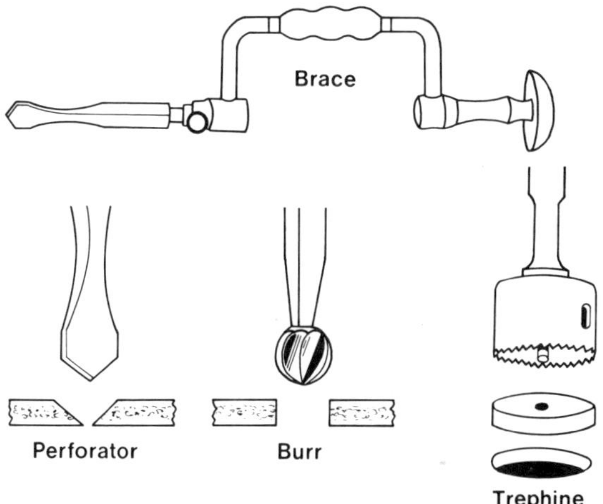

FIG. 19.4 Instruments used for burr and trephine holes.

converted into one with parallel sides by the use of a **burr.** The **dura mater** has to be opened by an **incision** with a knife. It is sometimes necessary to coagulate the cut edges with diathermy, and also the surface of the brain, before introducing the brain cannula. A **chronic subdural haematoma** is drained in this way after opening the sac which contains altered blood. This is washed out by irrigation with Ringer's solution at body temperature. It is usual to make at least two burr-holes for this purpose.

Air or radio-opaque contrast media may be introduced into either or both lateral brain ventricles through a cannula in order to make them visible in X-rays. This is called **ventriculography.** (**Air-encephalography** is another technique for showing the ventricles in X-rays. The air is introduced by lumbar or cisternal puncture in this method.) In very young babies a sharp needle can be passed into a lateral brain ventricle through the anterior fontanelle or coronal suture. Sometimes a hole in the skull may be made with a **twist drill** held in a special holder; in this case also, a sharp needle has to be used to penetrate the dura. Since the advent of computerised axial tomography (E.M.I. scan, see p.176), the need for ventriculography and air-encephalography has considerably decreased, although the latter is still an essential investigation for some conditions, including pituitary tumours which have extended in an upward direction.

A **trephine** is used to cut a circular disc of bone which can then be replaced at the end of the operation. It is sometimes used as an alternative to making an osteoplastic flap for intracranial procedures such as cortical biopsy, which can be performed through a relatively small opening.

Brain Incision and Tumour Excision

The 'skin' of the brain is the **pia mater,** and within this, the brain tissue has the consistency of soft jelly. Outside the pia mater, the **arachnoid mater** contains the surface cerebro-spinal fluid and blood vessels. In order to cut the brain, it is usual to grasp the pia and arachnoid and blood vessels with forceps, and to coagulate them with the diathermy before cutting with scissors. Once the surface has been penetrated, further blood vessels will be found at the bottom of the cerebral sulci, and these are treated in the same way. When the white matter is reached, the tissues are softer, the blood vessels are small, and it is usually cut with a fine metal sucker or by stroking with an instrument to both of which the diathermy is applied.

Diathermy

In addition to its use for **coagulating** blood vessels, the diathermy may be used for **cutting** firm tissues, in which case one electrode is joined to the cutting point on the **diathermy pencil** and the other to the neutral plate, which is usually on the patient's thigh. This technique is used for cutting muscles or separating them from bone. Some tough or large brain tumours, like certain firm meningiomas, may be cut with a **wire loop** and diathermy in order to remove them piecemeal. The **monopolar** arrangement, which has just been described, is generally used for coagulation and always for cutting, at least in the early stages of an operation, but there is a tendency for damage to occur beyond the point of the forceps due to spread of the intense heat. For this reason the monopolar method is not safe near the spinal cord or brain stem. This difficulty is avoided by using **bipolar** diathermy in which the current flows down one blade of a pair of forceps and up the other, the only electrical contact with the patient being through the tissue to be coagulated. This method is not used for cutting. For work on the tissues of the central nervous system the current has to be much less than would be used in other parts of the body (see Fig. 18.1).

Microsurgery

The **operating microscope** revolutionised the scope of ear, nose and throat surgery, and has now come to be applied to neurosurgery, especially for work on aneurysms, on the spinal cord and nerves, and for deep tumours and delicate structures. In addition to the advantages of magnification, the microscope provides its own illumination in the line of vision, which may be almost as important. It is possible for an assistant to see the view through the microscope by means of a separate eye-piece. It is also possible to take moving or still photographs. In place of the camera a small television tube can be fitted, which allows the operation to be transmitted by a closed circuit system to a television monitor. This enables the nurses assisting at the operation and any other observers to see what is going on, and the procedure can also be recorded on video tape. Special fine pointed and very delicate instruments are used.

Brain Abscess

Drainage of pus is obtained by **aspiration** through a cannula introduced through a burr-hole. The abscess cavity is usually outlined by a substance which is opaque to X-rays, such as 'Steripaque'. An **antibiotic** is also introduced. Aspiration is repeated when X-rays show the abscess is enlarging. The capsule may later be removed, if this can be done without further damage to the brain.

Aneurysms

Saccular aneurysms may be treated by placing a **clip** across the neck. These clips vary in size and design. They are left in position and prevent blood entering the aneurysm, the cavity of which is later obliterated by thrombosis. A silk **ligature** on the neck is sometimes used instead. If the **neck** of an aneurysmal sac is **broad** or **non-existent** it may make the application of a clip or ligature impossible, and the sac wall may then have to be reinforced by **wrapping** it with beaten muscle or cotton gauze. It is sometimes necessary to treat an aneurysm by reducing the pressure within the sac, by occluding one of the main vessels supplying it. Clearly this can only be done when there is an alternative route for the blood to supply the brain (Fig. 19.5).

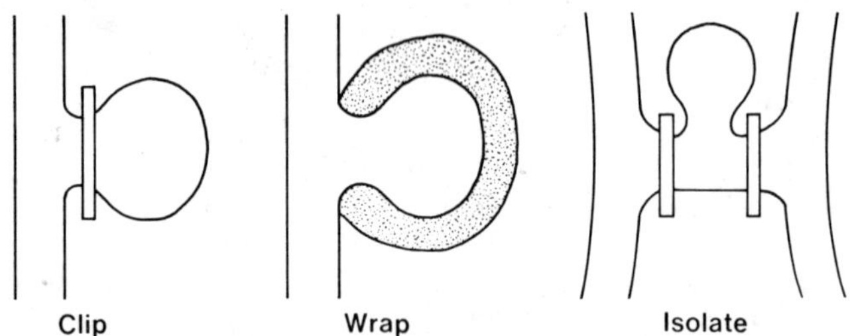

FIG. 19.5 Surgical treatment of cerebral aneurysms.

Shunts

The first successful shunt, by which is meant the use of a tube to transport cerebro-spinal fluid from one place to another, was the **ventriculo-cisternostomy** devised by Torkildsen (Fig. 19.6). In this operation a tube is placed between one or both lateral ventricles and the cisterna magna. It passes out from the ventricle through a burr-hole, and then beneath the scalp into the sub-occipital muscles, from where it re-enters the skull through another burr-hole or a small craniectomy. The end of the tube is placed well within the cisterna magna, thereby letting the cerebro-spinal fluid by-pass any obstruction in the foramen of Munro, third ventricle, aqueduct or fourth ventricle. No valves are used and there is no growth problem because

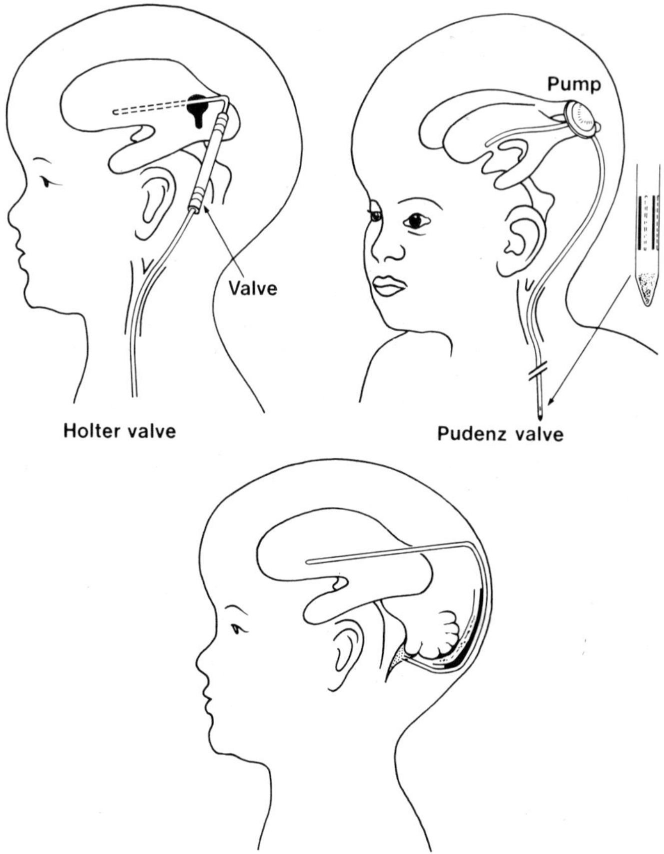

FIG. 19.6 Ventriculo-cisternostomy and two commonly used valves.

this part of the skull changes very little after the third or fourth year. Obviously, it is necessary for the remainder of the pathways through the basal cisterns and over the surface of the brain to be open, so that the cerebro-spinal fluid can reach the arachnoidal granulations beside the superior sagittal sinus, where most of it is absorbed. If there is an obstruction to the subarachnoid space, as there may be after meningitis, or in children with aqueduct stenosis in whom cerebro-spinal fluid has never flowed in sufficient quantity to open up all the pathways, the method of ventriculo-cisternostomy will not work. A valve type of shunt must then be used.

Tumours in the brain stem and some inflammatory processes tend to occlude the opening in the tentorium around the brain stem. If this is so, the cerebro-spinal fluid is only moved one stage further before its flow again becomes obstructed. Also, it is not a suitable method for very young babies, because the subarachnoid pathways over the brain are often undeveloped if there is an obstruction in the more proximal part of the cerebro-spinal fluid circulation. This is therefore a similar situation to the one that has just been described. Furthermore, the dura mater of the infant's posterior fossa contains large venous sinuses which mostly become obliterated after a few years; these may make the posterior fossa part of the operation very difficult. The present tendency is to use a valve system in another form of shunt, but the operation of ventriculo-cisternostomy still has a place in the treatment of aqueduct stenosis and some central space-occupying lesions over the age of three or four years.

Simple **drainage of a subdural sac** which will not respond to intermittent tapping is sometimes carried out by placing a tube between the interior of the sac and the **pleural cavity.** This tube passes through a burr-hole in the skull and then beneath the skin of the head and neck into the chest. The drainage is usually only required for a week or two, and the tube can be removed when the subdural haematoma no longer accumulates.

Valves

The two commonest types of valve are the **Spitz-Holter** and modifications of it, in which the valve mechanism lies under the scalp in the course of the tubing, and the **Pudenz** in which the valve is located at the outlet end of the tube (Fig. 19.6). In each case the valve is formed by a slit through which the cerebro-spinal fluid can pass in one direction only. Pressure in the opposite direction closes it. Shunts have been made between the ventricles and almost all the body cavities, but the only two receiving sites in common use at the present time are the **right atrium** of the heart, and the **peritoneal cavity.** In order to make a shunt between a **cerebral ventricle** and the heart, the tube passes from the ventricle through a burr-hole and then beneath the scalp and the skin of the neck into the **common facial vein,** which is a tributary of the **internal jugular vein.** It then passes within the vein into the **superior vena cava,** and so to the **right cardiac atrium.** In the case of a Holter type valve, the distal end of the tube is drawn out into a thin whip-like end. The valve itself has a compressible centre. This is a soft portion of silicone rubber tubing about 3 cm long in the valve mechanism. It can be made to act as a pump. Compression by pressure with a finger forces fluid through the tube into the heart and its subsequent release draws fluid from the ventricle. In this way, the function of the valve can be tested. The Pudenz valve, being at the end of the tube, lies in the heart in the case of a ventriculo-atrial shunt. In order to test the function of this type of valve a capsule is inserted in the system within the burr-hole in the skull. The capsule is not an essential part of the system, but can be pressed in order to find out if the tubes are patent, or to pump cerebro-spinal fluid from the ventricles.

All these shunts need to be revised from time to time if they are put into growing children, but in adults they usually function for years without revision. Sometimes a rather similar capsule to the one described is connected by a tube to a cerebral ventricle, but it has no distal outlet. This is a **reservoir** (Rickham or Ommaya) and it has no valve. It is used as a means of sampling the cerebro-spinal fluid or injecting substances when necessary. If need be, a reservoir can be joined to a shunt system.

Depressed Fractures

After head injury, any bone driven into the brain must be removed. It is also necessary to prevent pressure on the brain from indentation of the skull. Bone fragments may penetrate the dura and lacerate the underlying brain. Before removing them one must be able to deal with any haemorrhage that may be provoked. It is therefore sometimes necessary to remove bone around a depressed area in order to expose normal dura before doing this. The fragments can often be put back again. In the case of babies the skull is less brittle than in adults and it may merely be dented by a blow, so that the resulting depression can be pushed out by leverage through a burr-hole adjacent to the fracture without the need to expose it fully or undo it. If removed bone fragments cannot be replaced for fear of contamination and later infection of the wound, the treated depressed fracture will leave the patient with a defect in the bone. Unless this is quite small it should be repaired as described below.

Repair of skull defect. The missing bone is usually replaced with a **plastic inlay** of cold-curing polyester resin. The powder (**monomer**) is mixed with a special fluid (**catalyst**) to form a dough which hardens (**polymerisation**) in about 10 minutes. During the hardening process a considerable amount of heat is evolved, and so the final hardening must take place away from the tissues. The monomer and catalyst are very irritant to living cells and so the dough must be separated from them by plastic film or sheet of gutta percha during moulding. When hard, the new plate can be drilled, sawn, filed or bitten with rongeurs. Holes are usually drilled in the plate to allow fluid to pass through and fibrous tissue to grow across to unite the tissues on either side. Plates are sometimes made from sheet **tantalum** and other substances, but fashioning them into shape can be very difficult. **Bone grafts** may also be used to fill defects and are often taken from a rib, which can be split lengthwise to provide two pieces of bone with a suitable curvature.

Dural repair. Defects in the dura should be repaired if possible, particularly if they are related to fractured air sinuses, when they may cause **cerebro-spinal rhinorrhoea** and its complications. After the brain has been separated from a dural tear, and any spikes or fractured bone removed, openings into the air sinuses are covered by a **graft** of **fascia lata** from the thigh. This is laid on the brain side of the dura. If the graft is small, pericranium or temporalis fascia may be used instead. Defects over the cerebral hemispheres may be repaired with the same living materials or by using (freeze-dried) preserved human dura. Other substances, such as gelatin film or nylon film have been used but are less satisfactory.

Stereotactic Surgery

There are many varieties of stereotactic apparatus. All have the same function, which is to allow a fine instrument capable of destroying a small area of brain to be introduced through the skull to a target point. The targets depend on the part of the brain which is to be stimulated by an electric current, or from which electrical recordings are to be made, or which has to be destroyed in order to help the remainder of the brain to work more normally. They are plotted on air-encephalogram X-rays or on ventriculograms by measuring from structures which can be identified, such as the ventricles. The apparatus is always fixed temporarily to the skull by means of screws which penetrate the outer layer of the bone, and X-rays are taken to show the relationship of the apparatus to the target points from which measurements are to be made. Various atlases give 'map references' for the location of targets, and when the selected target is marked on X-ray films of the skull and apparatus, the lesion-maker is introduced and further X-rays are taken to confirm the accuracy of its placement. A recording of electrical activity through an electrode is sometimes used as an additional check. Small lesions from half to one centimetre in diameter, or less, are made by passing currents through an electrode, or by the use of a freezing method or a wire cutting-loop. The technique of stereotactic surgery was invented in order to study brain function in animals. It was applied to human surgery much later, but did not develop really significantly until it was applied to the treatment of **Parkinson's disease** about twenty-five years ago. Many different types of apparatus were then developed. However, it is now rarely that operations are done for this condition because of the newer types of drug therapy (l-dopa) which have improved medical treatment.

Stereotactic surgery is now used in the treatment of psychiatric patients (psychosurgery), certain types of intractable pain or movement disorder, and some operations for the treatment of epilepsy. The apparatus can also be used to obtain biopsies or to insert radioactive seeds.

Spinal Operations

It is usually necessary to remove the **spines** and **laminae** of several vertebrae in order to gain access to the vertebral canal within which the spinal cord and cauda equina lie. After doing a **laminectomy** the extradural space is exposed, allowing access to tumours or abscesses in this layer. If it is necessary to penetrate further, the dura is opened by a vertical midline incision and held open by sutures which cause tension on the dura and prevent haemorrhage from the extradural veins. These operations are done with the patient prone and on controlled respiration, thus reducing the amount of venous congestion. The spinal cord has to be handled **very delicately** and as little as possible when removing tumours that are compressing it from outside. Incisions may be made across part of the spinal cord (**chordotomy**) in order to divide pain pathways when other measures for the control of **pain** have failed. **Tumours** within the spinal cord can seldom be removed, but occasionally this may be done through a central incision (**myelotomy**). **Cysts** can be aspirated or drained, and spinal roots may be cut (**rhizotomy**). After operations of this sort, the dura mater is usually closed with interrupted silk sutures and made water-tight. It is sometimes necessary to leave it open and then the muscles have to be given an extra closure and no external drain may be used.

New surgical techniques are constantly being evolved or adapted from other branches of surgery, as in the case of the operating microscope. New discoveries of brain physiology allow surgeons to develop ways of offering help to patients for whom medical therapy has reached its limit. Then medical knowledge advances, and the same condition may return to the field of drug therapy. This emphasises the common ground of neurology and neurosurgery and the need to regard diseases of the nervous system as a single entity, which is neither surgical nor medical.

From the clinical history and examination the diagnosis is narrowed down to two or three possibilities. **Laboratory** and **X-ray studies** are now required to distinguish between them, or to confirm what has been the most probable diagnosis.

THE CEREBRO-SPINAL FLUID

Some neurological diseases produce clear-cut changes in the cerebro-spinal fluid of great value in diagnosis. In many others unfortunately the changes are too vague to be helpful. The fluid can be obtained by lumbar, cisternal, or ventricular puncture.

Lumbar Puncture (Fig. 20.1a) is the usual method employed. Because the meninges run further down the vertebral canal than does the cord itself, a sac containing C.S.F. is formed in the lumbar region into which a needle can be passed and fluid withdrawn, or substances injected, without damaging the cord. Normally the patient is positioned to lie on **one side,** with the back right at the **edge** of the bed and not leaning forwards. In order to separate the vertebral spines, the head and neck are **flexed** and the knees brought up towards the chin.

The lumbar skin is carefully cleaned with ether, spirit, or C.T.A.B., and the doctor may like to paint it with a further antiseptic. He will then select one of the spaces between the spines of L.2-S.1, towel off the area, and inject 2% procaine into the skin and subcutaneous tissues. The needle, which must contain the **correct stilette,** is passed in between the spinous processes into the lumbar sac (the **lumbar theca**). The stilette is withdrawn and a few drops of C.S.F. will escape if the needle is in the right place. Slight blood staining may be due to pricking a small skin vessel, but it will quickly clear. Heavy blood staining occurs if blood was already in the C.S.F. (e.g. in subarachnoid haemorrhage), or if a large vessel beyond the theca is entered. In the latter event the procedure will have to be repeated later.

C.S.F. pressure is measured by connecting a **manometer** to the needle by means of flexible rubber tubing. The nurse holds the manometer upright by its top, and the C.S.F. rises normally to a pressure of 100–150 mm (of C.S.F.). High pressure may be recorded if (a) a **frightened** patient holds himself tense—the nurse's attitude can help to prevent that; (b) an **obese** patient's knees compress the abdomen—the nurse will be asked gently to straighten the patient's legs; (c) there is **genuinely high pressure** inside the skull, due to

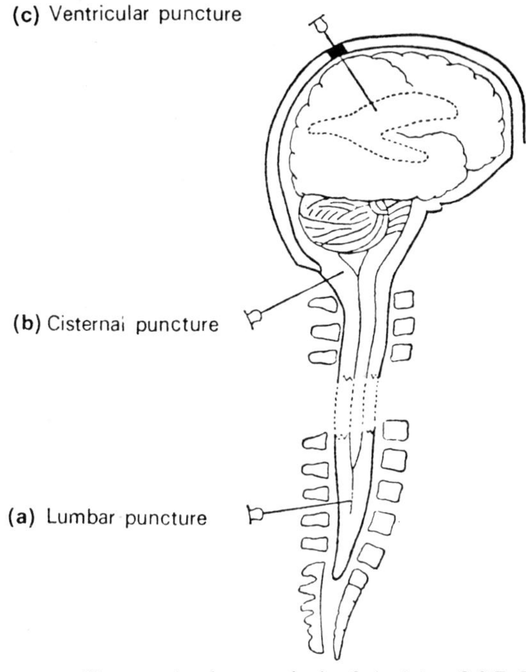

FIG. 20.1 Diagram to illustrate the three methods of obtaining C.S.F. In each case substances such as antibiotics, air, or opaque fluids for X-ray purposes, can be injected.

some unsuspected space-occupying lesion. If this is *known* to be present, e.g. from the presence of papilloedema, a lumbar puncture should not be carried out. Removal of the 'cushion' of C.S.F. from the lumbar region allows a brain tumour to force the brain downwards so that parts of the medulla and cerebellum are squeezed through the foramen magnum, forming a **cerebellar pressure cone.** This causes compression of the medulla, which may be fatal. At the same time a tentorial pressure cone (p. 46) forms for the same reason, and with the same result.

Queckenstedt Test. Compression of the **jugular veins** in the neck causes venous congestion inside the skull, and rise of C.S.F. pressure. This can be seen on the manometer, providing the C.S.F. pathways are not obstructed by, e.g. a spinal tumour. If the **block** is partial the C.S.F. may rise slowly, but fall barely at all—remember it is easier to squeeze toothpaste out of a tube than to put it back again.

The nurse presses with the **flat** of the hand on the **side** of the **neck** in front of the sternomastoid muscle, first on each side in turn, then both together. She must release the pressure quickly when told to do so.

Cisternal Puncture. The C.S.F. can be tapped in the **cisterna magna** (p. 19) by inserting a needle just beneath the base of the skull (Fig. 20.1b). This is of value if for some reason a lumbar puncture cannot be done, or if myodil is to be injected for descending myelography (see p. 176). The neck and **occipital region** must be **shaved** and the skin prepared as if for a surgical operation. The patient can sit upright, or lie on one side, with the head flexed forwards. The procedure, from the nurse's point of view, is similar to that of lumbar puncture, but pressures are not usually recorded. The needle is very close to the medulla, so that great care is required in positioning, steadying and reassuring the patient.

Ventricular Puncture can be carried out in states of **high intracranial pressure** without danger of pressure cone formation, for the C.S.F. is being removed from above the danger area. It is a surgical procedure, carried out in the theatre. The **skull** is **shaved** and the skin prepared. Local anaesthetic is injected into the skin and subcutaneous tissues, a small incision made, and a hole (a **burr-hole**) drilled into the skull. A needle is then passed through the brain into one of the lateral ventricles (Fig. 20.1c). Ventricular puncture is usually carried out either as part of the X-ray process of **ventriculography** (p. 174), or as an **emergency** measure to reduce a sudden rise in intracranial pressure, or to introduce antibiotics when lumbar puncture is not advisable.

Collection of the Fluid

About 8 ml of the C.S.F. is collected and inspected at once. A **cloudy C.S.F.** (if the glassware is clean) means a raised cell count; a **red C.S.F.** means blood; a **yellow** or xanthochromic **C.S.F.** means either old blood, or a very high protein. If blood is present the fluid is collected in two tubes, and if the blood comes from a superficial vessel, the second tube will be clear. If still bloodstained it ought to be **centrifuged** at once, for a yellow supernatant fluid will mean the blood was there before the puncture. The fluid must not stand overnight on the ward. For analysis, especially of cells and sugar, to be reliable, it must be sent to the laboratory **at once.** Therefore, arrange punctures **early** in the day. The fluid is examined for **cells, protein, W.R.,** and **Lange curve,** and sometimes for sugar and chlorides. A table showing the main abnormalities is given on p. 194.

The nurse can allay much of the patient's anxiety about these procedures by regarding them as of routine nature, similar to blood tests, and by trying to prevent other patients from increasing this anxiety by lurid and inaccurate accounts of their own experiences.

THE BLOOD AND URINE

Neurological symptoms are often due to involvement of the nervous system by a disease which affects many organs, and the clue to its nature may come from examination of body fluids other than the C.S.F. In all cases a full blood-count, a sedimentation rate, and a W.R. should be carried out, and the urine should be tested for albumin, sugar, cells and casts. The possible value of these investigations is given in the tables on pp. 193–196.

FAECES

The stools are examined for occult blood while searching for a possible primary intestinal tumour if metastases are suspected. Excessive fat excretion is looked for in cases of obscure polyneuropathy, for steatorrhoea may cause serious vitamin deficiency. If parasitic infestation is possible, the worm or its eggs may be found. In virus diseases of the nervous system, especially poliomyelitis, the virus may be isolated from the faeces or urine.

X-RAYS

Nervous tissue is not opaque to ordinary X-rays, therefore this type of investigation would be useless if it were not that certain diseases produce (a) changes in the skull or spine which can be shown by **plain** or **straight** X-rays; or (b) alterations in the normal shape or position of the **ventricles** or **blood-vessels** which can be made visible by injecting some substance into them. These are called **contrast studies,** and the contrast may be produced by something denser than its surroundings, e.g. myodil in **myelography,** or a variety of opaque substances in **arteriography**—or by air, which is less dense than brain tissue, and is used in **pneumoencephalography** and **ventriculography.**

Since the last edition of this book was published a dramatic new development has revolutionised neurological diagnosis within the field of neuroradiology. Bearing the somewhat forbidding title of **Computerised Axial Tomography** and carried out by a very expensive machine popularly known as the **E.M.I. scanner**, this technique is rapidly making some of the well established methods of investigation out of date. However, not every centre is able to acquire one of these highly expensive machines, and a description will therefore be given of the more familiar methods of neuroradiological investigation first.

Straight X-rays

These obviously will show fractures or dislocations of the skull and spine, or degenerative bony changes such as spondylosis. Space-occupying lesions can, however, also be suspected if there is erosion of bone, enlargement of nerve foramina (neurofibromas), erosion of the sella turcica (a sign of high intracranial pressure), enlargement of the sella (pituitary tumour), and displacement of the pineal, which is often calcified and therefore visible and should lie exactly in the midline.

The purpose of contrast studies is to locate the lesion accurately, if possible to determine its nature, and to show types of lesion which do not alter the bone structure.

Pneumoencephalography (or Air-encephalography)

The aim of this procedure is to show up the ventricles and subarachnoid spaces. The patient sits upright with his head suitably positioned in the X-ray machine, a lumbar (or occasionally cisternal) puncture is performed, and about 30 ml of air are slowly injected. The air travels up into the ventricles and over the surface of the brain. By taking pictures with the head in various positions, the size, shape and position of the **ventricles** and **subarachnoid spaces** can be seen, and it is possible to show if they are **displaced** by tumours, or **enlarged** by atrophy.

Ventriculography

Because of the danger of pressure cone (p. 46), lumbar air-encephalography is unsafe in high intracranial pressure, but if air is introduced directly into the ventricles through a burr-hole, this danger is avoided. The position of a tumour can be shown by distortion or displacement of the lateral ventricles, and the air can then be made to run through the aqueduct and IVth ventricle to show any obstruction or displacement by brain stem or posterior fossa tumours. In the latter event, to give even clearer pictures, myodil is sometimes introduced as well.

Arteriography

Blood vessels cannot normally be seen on X-rays, but by injecting an **opaque dye** into the **carotid** or **vertebral** arteries with the patient lying on the X-ray table, and then taking several photographs within a few **seconds,** first the cerebral arteries, then the capillaries, and finally the veins, can be clearly shown.

An experienced arteriographer can pass a needle directly through the skin into the artery under local or general anaesthesia. For the vertebral arteries a fine catheter is often passed into the femoral artery and threaded up through the aorta, under X-ray screen control, until the tip lies in the subclavian artery at the opening of the vertebral artery. Dye is then injected through the catheter.

The normal appearance and position of blood vessels have now been accurately worked out and arteriography can show (a) **displacement** of vessels by a tumour, cyst, or haematoma; (b) the sac of an **aneurysm,** or the mass of vessels in an **angioma**; (c) abnormal vessels in a **tumour,** which may give a pattern characteristic of a particular type of tumour (especially the benign **meningiomas** and the very malignant **glioblastomas**); and (d) absence of a vessel due to **thrombosis**; or narrowing due to **atheroma.**

Arteriography is a safe procedure in high intracranial pressure, does not require burr-holes, and may give a diagnosis immediately.

Echo-Encephalography

If **ultrasonic waves** are passed through the skull from one side to the other they bounce back from certain structures, including those which should be situated in exactly the **midline.** These waves can be recorded on a small television screen, and it can be seen if these midline structures are displaced to one side, e.g. by a tumour or haematoma. It is a simple, harmless and painless procedure which can be carried out in the out-patient department, and if positive points to a **space-occupying lesion.**

Isotope Encephalography (or Brain Scanning)

Brain scanning is now an invaluable aid to diagnosis. A small and quite harmless dose of a **radioactive compound** is injected intravenously, and the **isotope** is taken up by **cerebral tumours** or areas of damaged brain (such as an **infarct**), but not by normal brain tissue. A complicated piece of apparatus automatically scans the skull and photographs on X-ray plates any areas where there is abnormal concentration of the isotope. Again an out-patient investigation, this can be safely used on any adult, with the exception of pregnant women, and may save a number of admissions to hospital for the much more expensive and less comfortable arteriograms, or air-encephalograms. It is particularly helpful in picking up **meningiomas** and multiple tumours such as **metastases.**

Computerised Axial Tomography (C.A.T. Scanning)

The process of C.A.T. scanning, using X-rays alone, depends upon the fact that different tissues, e.g. bone, brain, tumour tissue, or fluid absorb X-rays to different degrees. These different degrees can be measured and photographed by the scanner so that the bones of the skull, the shape and position of the ventricles, and the presence of tumours, cysts, haemorrhages and infarcts are shown with a clarity almost as if one were looking at a pathological specimen. Intravenous injection of certain contrast media (which enhance abnormalities) and newer methods of displaying the results enable more detail to be seen.

As this method becomes widely available it is likely that air-encephalography and echo-encephalography will disappear; arteriography will be strikingly reduced and isotope scanning may become restricted to use in research. Many craniotomies and cerebral biopsies for diagnostic purposes will be unnecessary. The risk to the patient is negligible; the discomfort slight; children can be examined as well as adults; there is only need for anaesthesia if the patient is unable to co-operate, e.g. babies and young children. However, only a limited number of examinations can be carried out in the space and time available and costs of installation and maintenance are high. As accuracy improves the saving in in-patient bed costs may well offset these disadvantages and no doubt newer more economical techniques will be developed in time. The spinal canal, spinal cord and other parts of the body can already be subject to this type of examination using the whole body scanner. This one investigation has been the greatest advance in neurological diagnosis in two generations.

Myelography

A spinal tumour or prolapsed disc causes **complete** or **partial block** to the flow of C.S.F. This may be shown by the Queckenstedt test, but its exact site can only be determined by introducing an opaque substance, such as **myodil,** through a lumbar puncture needle into the **spinal theca.** The patient sits up until he is taken to the X-ray table, where he is **tilted** up and down under a viewing screen. Indentations or obstruction to the myodil can then be photographed. If a block is complete from below, its upper end can be shown by running myodil down from the cisterna magna. In some cases air is used instead of myodil—this may be particularly useful in showing the cord itself in e.g. syringomyelia. At myelography a **marker** is often strapped on the skin at the level of the block to guide the surgeon when making his incision. Any nurse who carelessly removes this will be very unpopular indeed!

ELECTROENCEPHALOGRAPHY

The living brain is constantly discharging small **electrical waves** which can be picked up from the surface of the head, magnified and recorded on paper. The machine which does this is called an **electroencephalograph,** or **E.E.G.,** and the tracing it produces is an **electroencephalogram.**

Little **electrodes** are held on to the scalp, either by a hair net, or by collodion, and spaced out to cover the whole skull. These are connected to the recording **pens,** and the controls of the machine allow tracings to be made on moving paper from any combination of these electrodes.

From the occipital region, when the eyes are shut, there are normally regular runs of waves called the **alpha rhythm** (Fig. 20.2). In other areas a slower rhythm called **theta** may appear. In abnormal tracings theta activity is excessive and **slower** waves still,

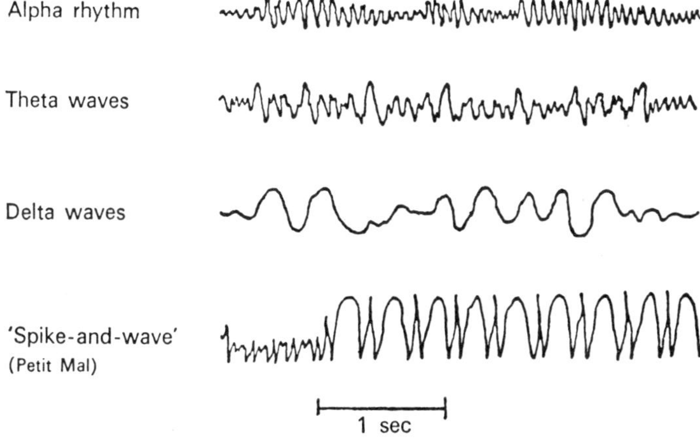

FIG. 20.2 Different types of E.E.G. waves.

called **delta,** are seen. Over brain containing (say) a tumour, slow waves may be seen coming from one area only, and there is said to be **focal discharge** from that area. This helps in locating a lesion, but as many different lesions produce the same type of abnormality, one cannot say exactly what the lesion is.

In epileptic patients the E.E.G. may show abnormalities **in between** the fits. This is not always so, however, so that it cannot prove that a patient has *not* got epilepsy. To make it more difficult, some quite normal people have abnormal waves similar to those seen in known epileptics. They may be the carriers of the epileptic tendency, but it does not mean they are themselves epileptics.

It will be understood, therefore, that the E.E.G. can only be used to *support* the clinical diagnosis, and it must not be expected to *make* one.

Petit mal epilepsy, however, shows runs of a very characteristic abnormality; a high voltage sharp wave followed by a large slow wave three times a second—the so-called **spike-and-wave** (Fig. 20.2).

If abnormalities are too slight to be of value, they may be made more definite by several means, (a) by making the patient breathe deeply for 3 minutes (hyperventilation or **overbreathing**); (b) by sending him to **sleep** by the use of a barbiturate; (c) giving enough of a **stimulant** (Metrazol) to produce a sub-clinical fit, i.e. an epileptic discharge shown on the E.E.G. but not producing a convulsion.

In **temporal lobe epilepsy** the abnormal discharges may come from underneath the brain, far away from the scalp. Special needles, called **sphenoidal electrodes,** can be passed through the malar region to lie below the sphenoidal bones, very near the temporal lobes, and the abnormal waves recorded from there.

At times a surgeon may wish to take tracings **directly** from the **brain** itself in the operating theatre. This is done with special electrodes, using the same E.E.G. machine, but the procedure is called **electrocorticography.** The site of a small lesion, e.g. a scar, may thus be located very accurately and then excised.

ELECTROMYOGRAPHY

The **electromyograph** (E.M.G.) records electrical **discharges** given off in **muscle** fibres. Normally there are none at rest, but they become profuse when the muscle contracts. Fine electrodes are either attached to the skin, or introduced into the muscle itself, and the waves are seen on a little television **screen** (a cathode-ray oscilloscope) and at the same time photographed on a moving **film,** so that they can be studied later. By different wave patterns the E.M.G. helps to distinguish between a muscle that is weak and wasted because its nerve supply is damaged, i.e. it is de-nervated, and one whose disease is in the muscle itself, e.g. muscular dystrophy.

It can also be used to measure the speed with which an electrical stimulus travels from some point on a nerve to the muscle that that nerve supplies. This is called the **nerve conduction time** and it may be delayed by damage to the nerve along its course.

Both E.E.G. and E.M.G. are wonderful instruments, but they are not miraculous, and are often unreliable, especially the E.E.G. in epilepsy. They are not computers which will make the diagnosis for the doctor, and neither doctor, nor nurse, should ever allow the patient to think that they will.

21 *SOME ESSENTIAL PRINCIPLES OF NEUROLOGICAL NURSING*

Perhaps the most remarkable feature of the nervous system is its capacity to recover, often completely, from what has appeared to be a state of total loss of function. Though this degree of recovery may not always take place, the nursing approach to acute neurological problems must assume that it will. The whole basis of treatment must therefore be to ensure that if and when recovery occurs the patient's body is in the right physical condition to take advantage of it. Patients unable to breathe or swallow properly must not be allowed to suffocate or choke. Restless patients must not injure themselves. Paralysed patients must not develop bed sores, or lung collapse, or urinary infection. Comatose patients must not starve or become dehydrated, and those with weak or paralysed limbs must not develop stiff joints in faulty positions so that when strength returns they are too deformed to be useful. There is a lot of nursing to be done and the responsibility is heavy, but as the nervous system can only respond to disease in certain ways, the number of different nursing situations to be faced is not large, even if the number of possible diseases is.

The Comatose Patient

The special problems in coma arise from the patient's inability to swallow, cough, feed himself, and control the bladder and bowels. If such a patient is nursed or transported simply lying flat, there is constant danger of tracheal obstruction from the tongue falling backwards, or from inhaled saliva, mucus, or vomit.

Nursing should be carried out in the **semi-prone position,** the head turned to one side so that the mouth and nostrils are not obstructed by the pillow, the legs protected, by pillows, from pressing on each other, and the foot of the bed raised so that secretions will drain into the pharynx rather than the lungs. An electrically driven sucker fitted with a firm catheter must be kept by the bed, the pharynx sucked out at regular intervals throughout the day, and immediately there is any sign of 'bubbling', cyanosis, or respiratory distress. If this does not relieve breathing difficulty the foot of the bed should be raised even further and medical help summoned.

If a **clear airway** is not obtained a tracheostomy may be necessary, and this should be done too early rather than too late. Suction of the trachea can then be carried out with much greater ease and efficiency through the tracheostomy tube. If there is pulmonary collapse, bronchoscopy may be required for efficient suction.

Careful watch is kept on the **level of consciousness.** This is assessed by the response to unpleasant stimuli, pressure on the supraorbital notch or firm rubbing on the sternum. Any deepening of coma must be reported at once.

The size and reaction of the **pupils** are watched—pupillary dilation or a change from normal reaction to no reaction must be reported at once.

The **pulse rate** must be recorded—in a head injury or cranial operation every $\frac{1}{4}$ hour at first. Any marked slowing or sudden acceleration must be reported.

These could all be signs of increasing intracranial pressure, and might need surgical interference. No nurse will be criticised for being over cautious in this respect.

If increasing intracranial pressure is suspected from increasing headache, vomiting, deepening coma and slowing of the pulse, several emergency procedures are available.

At one time **hypertonic solutions** given intravenously were the most effective measures available, and **urea, mannitol** or 50% **sucrose** were regularly used. They were dangerous in the presence or renal failure and highly corrosive to veins. Enemata of magnesium sulphate was an even older but sometimes effective method. **Mannitol** is still used but nowadays **steroids** are preferred, being easy to administer either by injection or orally; their dosage is better controlled; and they are effective in reducing swelling of brain tissue. **Dexamethazone** and **betamethazone** are in most common usage. These have the advantage of being able to be continued orally after the acute phase has settled and so avoid a back-lash effect when the effect of the initial injections has worn off.

Lumbar puncture should **never** be used to reduce acute increase of intracranial pressure, but the surgeon may wish to tap the ventricles through burr-holes and may even wish to leave a ventricular drain until more detailed surgical correction of the condition is possible.

A comatose patient's position must be changed at least every two hours, and the same care given to the skin as in a paraplegic (p. 182).

No attempt should be made to feed an unconscious or semiconscious patient by mouth—this may prove fatal. In the early stages an **intravenous drip** may be necessary to provide adequate fluid, but for the longer term a **tube** is passed through the nostril into the stomach, and small but frequent feeds of milk, protein, and vitamin concentrate given at regular intervals throughout the day.

The **bladder** must be palpated every 4 hours, even if the patient is incontinent, for over distension can cause renal damage and bladder rupture. The **bowels** can be cared for by enemas every third or fourth day. The **mouth** must be cleaned several times each day and great care taken of the **conjunctivae.**

A patient coming out of coma is often restless and sometimes violent. This may be due to bladder discomfort, or some other unpleasant sensation not fully appreciated. **Padded cot-sides** and restraining nets may both be required temporarily, and sedation may be ordered by the medical staff, varying according to the cause of the coma.

The Hemiplegic Patient

Hemiplegic limbs are often flaccid at first, and may lie in so bad a position that when spasticity later develops the muscle **contracture** that accompanies it may fix joints in useless postures. The patient must not be allowed to slump to the paralysed side. He should be well supported by pillows, the head maintained straight. **Pillows** are also placed under the arm so that the shoulder is abducted, and the elbow slightly flexed. The wrist should be held in dorsiflexion by a light **cock-up splint** applied to the forearm. Though the knees should be supported they should not be flexed, and the feet must be held in dorsiflexion by **sandbags,** the weight of the bedclothes being taken off by a **cradle.** The reason for this is that as paralysis recovers a neglected arm is pulled inwards at the shoulder, the wrist drops, the knees flex, and the foot drops. These deformities can develop quite quickly, and are exceedingly difficult to overcome. For the same reason, each joint should be moved through its **full range** twice each day, even after some return of power is evident. This especially applies to the shoulder, for a 'frozen shoulder' is a frequent and very painful complication of a neglected hemiplegia.

There is particular danger in a paralysed leg of thrombosis developing in the deep veins; for this reason the patient is mobilised as quickly as possible and if this is not possible the calves must be carefully examined each day for swelling or tenderness, and for pain on dorsiflexing the foot. The great danger lies not so much in the leg but in a clot detaching itself and forming an embolism which lodges in the lungs. Pulmonary embolism is a common cause of sudden death in bedridden or post-operative patients and can be prevented by correct use of anticoagulants.

The nurse is strongly recommended to read the excellently illustrated articles on passive movements and limb positioning in the *Nursing Times* of 1962 (Sept. 28, p. 1232; Oct. 5, p. 1261; Oct. 12, p. 1289).

The Paraplegic Patient

Paralysis of both legs is usually accompanied by loss of skin sensation and urinary control. There are, therefore, a number of problems to be faced. An acute paraplegia is often flaccid at first, but as with hemiplegia, spasticity and a tendency to muscle contracture gradually develops, the joints may become flexed and fixed, and painful **flexor** and **extensor spasms** occur.

The position of the limbs is again important. The knees must be kept almost straight, and the feet supported in dorsiflexion. Flexed knees and dropped feet are severe disabilities to an otherwise recovered patient.

With loss of sensation the danger of **bed sores** is acute. **Bony prominences** must be well protected and pressure evenly distributed. The **heels** should be kept off the bed by placing a pillow under the **calves**—never by rings under the heels. The patient should be nursed on a sorbo-rubber, or foam-rubber mattress, or on a 'ripple' bed. He should spend a high proportion of the time in the **prone** position, the pillows being so arranged that there is no pressure on the elbows, iliac spines, knees or the dorsum of the feet. Patients will not like this, and the purpose of it must be vividly explained to them.

The **skin** should be treated twice daily with gentle massage by a lubricated hand over all the pressure areas. Vigorous rubbing may abrade the skin and increase the chance of bedsores. The skin should be sprayed with **silicone** to protect it against moisture. All wrinkles must be smoothed out of bed-clothes, and the patient must never be allowed to lie in a wet bed. Hot water bottles must not be placed in the bed, no matter how well they are protected. When the patient is turned or moved there must be enough people present to ensure that he is lifted and not dragged.

Care of the **bladder** is dealt with separately below. It is better for the bowels to be somewhat constipated, enemas being given every third day preceded by instillation of olive oil if faeces become very hard.

Passive full movements of each joint should be carried out daily. In spastic paraplegia flexor spasms are usually troublesome. They are triggered off by touching, and exaggerated by urinary infection. Clothes should be arranged to avoid stimulating these spasms, and attempts will be made to reduce spasticity and to reduce sensitivity by muscle relaxants and sedatives.

For the established paraplegic, life can be made easier by use of the various **hoists** which are available from local authorities, the British Red Cross, or privately. Patients can be raised for bed-making, transferred to a chair or commode, to a bath, or even to a car, with minimum effort. If it is evident that the paraplegia will be permanent, rehabilitation of the special type available at **paraplegic centres** should be started from the earliest possible moment. The degree of mobility and independence achieved by these measures can be highly rewarding.

The Bladder

A patient may have **incontinence** of urine, **retention** of urine, or retention of urine with **overflow incontinence,** the bladder being so over filled that small amounts dribble away incessantly. In any comatose or paraplegic patient the **urinary output** must be watched, charted if possible, and the bladder must be **palpated** twice daily in order to detect overdistension, for the patient may be quite unaware of this.

If the bladder becomes distended, or retention has been present for more than 8 hours, a **catheter** should be passed with as strict an **aseptic technique** as any surgical operation—neurological patients very easily develop troublesome urinary infections. For this reason repeated catheterisation should be avoided if possible. It is best to leave in a fine catheter and have this connected to a plastic urine receptacle. Continuous drainage should not be allowed, however, for in neurological patients the bladder may eventually become small and permanently contracted. The tube should be clipped and released every three or four hours to allow the bladder to be filled and emptied in as near normal a manner as possible. Samples of urine are examined in the bacteriology laboratory and through the same tube the bladder can be irrigated with an antiseptic solution chosen according to the infection present. The appropriate antibiotics will be given by mouth at the same time. The preparation used will be determined by culturing the organisms from the urine and finding to which antibiotic or sulphonamide they are most susceptible. Tidal drainage was once commonly used and always the bane of a nurse's life as the apparatus was temperamental in the extreme and flooded wards were common. This is now rarely employed and the technique will not be described in this edition.

For **incontinence** it is essential to place an **indwelling catheter** at once. A series of wet beds is certain sooner or later to cause damage to the skin and encourage bed sores. This again can be released at intervals. Continuous drainage into a bottle is to be avoided, for this encourages the bladder to remain in a small contracted state and eventually to become capable of holding small quantities only.

For **permanent retention** attempts are made to encourage the **automatic bladder.** For a period of 10–14 days the catheter is released at exact intervals of four hours. It is then removed and at the same exact intervals the patient tries to pass urine himself, aided by manual compression of the abdomen and injections of carbachol. By perseverence many patients are able to empty their bladders and remain dry between these regular intervals. For permanent incontinence a **portable urinal** is necessary. These are only partially satisfactory and the female models are barely that. They are worn strapped to the inside of the thigh and give a degree of mobility otherwise denied to the patient. Though not widely used yet, an apparatus can be implanted to stimulate the bladder to contract in response to a radio or electrical signal given by the patient. Research into this technique is making considerable progress.

Bed Sores

If care of the skin has been adequate these should not develop. If they do they need urgent treatment, for in an emaciated patient, or particularly in one who has **loss of sensation,** they enlarge rapidly and necrotic infected **sloughs** soon form. **The patient must be nursed in such a way that he does not rest on the sores.** This may mean constant nursing in the prone position despite all protests; otherwise treatment will fail. **Swabs** should be taken from the surface and depths of the sore and **cultures** prepared of any infecting organism. Dressings are carried out twice daily with eusol or flavine, and the surface is sprayed with the antibiotic to which the organism is sensitive. The aim being to produce a clean granulating surface, sloughs must be carefully cleaned off. **Antibiotics** may be given systematically and protein loss and anaemia is corrected by a **high protein diet, protein concentrates,** and **blood transfusion. Anabolic steroids** may be added with benefit. A great recent advance has been the application to a sore of a preparation containing minute spheres which absorb both exudate and bacteria and allow the granulation tissue to form. If the patient co-operates well and a clean sore is obtained, excision and suture, or skin grafting may become possible. Remember, however, no sore will heal, whatever the treatment, if the pressure of the body weight rests upon it.

Respiratory Paralysis

If there is danger of respiratory muscle paralysis, i.e. in cases of poliomyelitis, polyneuritis, or lesions high in the cervical region, the **rate** and **depths** of respiration, and the patient's **colour** must be carefully watched. By testing how far they can count in one breath their respiratory capacity can be tested and progressive difficulty detected. There is a growing tendency for patients with respiratory failure to be transferred to a respiratory unit where highly trained staff are available to give the complex and constant care required.

Artificial respiration is normally carried out either by the tank respirators, or by intermittent positive pressure. Modern **tank respirators,** being hinged at the foot and opening like a crocodile's jaws, are much easier to put the patient into and, having large ports at the sides, make nursing care more practicable than was the case formerly. **Positive pressure** is now usually given in conjunction with tracheostomy, the pump being connected to the tracheostomy tube and the need to enclose the patient in a box is avoided. This makes nursing care infinitely easier.

Respiratory paralysis is frequently accompanied by paralysis of **swallowing** and of the palate and pharynx. Such cases must be nursed in the **head-down** position so that secretions drain into the tonsillar region and can be sucked out. This applies whether in a tank or on positive pressure, but with the tracheostomy, of course, much more efficient tracheal suction is possible.

The problem of nursing a case of respiratory failure is a very large one, too large to be dealt with in this chapter, and the reader is strongly recommended to the detailed account given in the book *Neurological Nursing* by Dr. John Marshall (Blackwell).

It is vital for the nurse to remember that dramatic though the failure to breathe may be, the patient still needs the same care of skin, bladder and positioning of limbs as in any other case of widespread paralysis.

22 *THE NURSE'S SPECIAL RESPONSIBILITY IN NEUROLOGY*

Neurologists and neurosurgeons depend a great deal on the nursing staff in the diagnosis as well as the management of their cases. The nurse, for instance, sees a lot more of the relatives and friends, who often give vital clues. Diagnostic symptoms and signs are often present for a short time only and may have disappeared by the time a doctor is available, and it is the nurse who has the opportunity of observing them. She must know what information from these sources is likely to be of value to the doctor. As she must also try to help patients to face the problems of the future, she should know which are the wisest and kindest answers to the questions they most frequently ask.

ON ADMISSION

The History from the Relatives

Ideally the doctor should see the relatives of every patient on admission. This may not always be possible immediately, and as the relatives may have far to travel, the nurse admitting the patient should make a note of details which the patient may not be able to give. This is absolutely essential when the patient is (a) admitted in **stupor** or **coma,** (b) **confused, disorientated,** or suffering from **defective memory,** (c) suffers from **epilepsy** or attacks of **loss of consciousness,** and (d) is a **child.** Taking each in turn, the medical staff will want to know the details listed below:

The Comatose Patient

(a) How long has he been unconscious?
(b) Were there any symptoms beforehand, especially headache, vomiting, or convulsions; if so, for how long?
(c) Was there any injury prior to the coma?
(d) Did the patient become unconscious suddenly or gradually; and if gradually, over how long?
(e) Has this happened before; if so, how many times?
(f) Is there any family history of attacks of loss of consciousness?
(g) Was the patient on any drugs, or did he have access to drugs; what were they?
(h) Has there been any emotional trouble at home, at work, etc.?

Attacks of Loss of Consciousness

These details should be obtained from the patient, the relatives, or a witness of an attack:
(a) At what age did attacks start?
(b) How often do they occur and when was the last?
(c) Is there any warning, and if so, what is it like?

(d) Does the patient lose consciousness completely?
(e) What happens during an attack? Are there any convulsions or twitching of arms or legs; are the eyes shut or open; do they roll or turn upwards; or does the patient simply lie completely still?
(f) If there are convulsions, can one recognise a tonic and clonic phase, and is one side or one part of the body only or principally affected?
(g) Is there tongue-biting or incontinence?
(h) What is the patient's colour?
(i) On recovery is there any confusion, abnormal behaviour, paralysis?
(j) How long do the various stages last?
(k) Is there any history of birth injury, head injury, serious cerebral illness?
(l) Is there any family history of epilepsy, or loss of consciousness?
(m) Is the patient on any drugs; has he been taking them regularly?

Loss of Memory, Confusion, Disorientation

(a) How long has this been present?
(b) Did it come on suddenly, or gradually?
(c) Was there any preceding illness or injury?
(d) Does it vary at all?
(e) Is it getting worse or better?
(f) Does he know who he is, where he is, who his wife and children are?
(g) Is the memory loss for recent events, distant events, or both? For names of people; of things; or both?
(h) Does he interest himself in papers, radio, T.V.?
(i) Does he know his way about the house, around the streets, in his home?

Children

(a) How many children in the family; this child's position?
(b) Any difficulties at birth, after birth, in infancy?
(c) Any maternal illness during pregnancy?
(d) At what age did the child sit up, stand, walk, talk, read?
(e) Any deterioration recently in any of these.
(f) Any so-called 'febrile' or 'teething' convulsions.
(g) What past illnesses; any particularly serious ones?
(h) Any past accidents or injuries?
(i) If adopted or illegitimate, any knowledge of parent's medical history?
(j) Are the blood groups, especially Rh, known?
(k) Progress at school; age of other classmates.
(l) Any of the other details previously listed which apply in this particular case?

It is also advisable to have the parent's consent to obtaining a report from the school if this should be thought necessary.

OBSERVATIONS IN THE WARD

Any change in the patient's physical condition or behaviour must be observed and reported promptly and accurately. Such changes may be temporary—as when the patient has a fit, or progressive—as when a patient becomes increasingly drowsy, or increasingly paralysed.

In the case of fits or periods of confused or disordered behaviour, the details mentioned above must be noted at first hand. The corneal reflexes, the reaction of the pupils, the plantar reflexes and the strength of the limbs on recovery should all be tested and the results written down. If a paralysis develops, the side affected and the extent is noted, the speed of development, the length of time it lasts and the presence of any other symptoms, such as headache, vomiting, visual or speech disturbance, loss of consciousness, or convulsions.

It is not enough just to fill in a form stating that the patient had a fit; think what the doctor (who may not arrive until it is all over) wants to know. This especially applies to the side affected by convulsions or any subsequent paralysis.

Speech Disturbances

The speed of onset, and the presence of other symptoms such as a fit, headache, or hemiparesis, are noted, and an attempt should be made to decide if the defect is dysphasia or dysarthria (p. 41).

Incontinence

(a) Is the patient incontinent of both urine and faeces?
(b) Is there any loss of consciousness at this time?
(c) Is it a constant dribble, or a sudden evacuation of the bladder?
(d) If a dribble, palpate the bladder. Is it due to overflow from over distension?
(e) If a full evacuation, is the patient able to ask for and use the bedpan normally at other times, or is he too lethargic to do so?

The urinary output and fluid intake should always be noted and measured if it appears unusually large (diabetes insipidus), or unusually small.

The Pupils

Pay particular attention to the size and reactions of the pupils when any deterioration takes place in a patient's condition. Temporary failure to react to light on both sides is common during a fit, but if one pupil begins to dilate this is usually a serious sign (see p. 46), and the nurse may be the first to detect it.

QUESTIONS AND ANSWERS

Many patients entering a neurological ward want reassurance on many points that are worrying them, and feeling that doctors are too busy to spare the time, they often turn to the nurses for help. They fear that neurological and mental disease are the same, and that a neurological unit is a thinly disguised mental hospital. They have heard lurid, third-hand accounts of the 'horrors' of investigations and think an E.E.G. is a form of E.C.T. (electroconvulsive therapy), and that a brain operation must inevitably result in mental deterioration.

Be guided by the medical staff in the approach to each patient, but frankness and honesty about the nature and purpose of the tests, and which parts may be unpleasant and which not, usually go a long way towards settling the patient's mind. Questions regarding the future are many, but those which recur with greatest frequency are discussed below. If the nurse is to give answers to these, she must be confident her answers will be correct.

In Epilepsy

How long must I take this treatment? Never say 'not long'. Patients must realise that treatment must be absolutely regular until there has been no trace of a fit for at least three years and perhaps longer. It must never be stopped without medical advice. In the early stages success with treatment is an indication for continuing it rather than stopping it.

Will it cure me? It will not *cure* the underlying epileptic tendency, but it has an excellent chance, though not a certainty, of preventing that tendency from producing any symptoms, i.e. fits. The epileptic tendency usually gets less with age, so that successful control in early years may result in permanent freedom.

Is there any danger of becoming a mental case? If the epilepsy is not due to progressive disease of the brain, the answer is 'No'.

What about driving? It is *illegal* for an epileptic still subject to fits to drive. Unfortunately many patients ignore this and expose themselves and others to great danger. As regards the hope of driving in the future, the law is now quite clear about this. A patient must have been free of all traces of a fit for a minimum period of three years before he is allowed to drive. The only exception to this is that some patients have their fits only while asleep at night, but this must have been shown to be true for a minimum period of three years before the licensing authorities will accept the fits as 'purely nocturnal'. It must be realised that anyone advising an epileptic 'not to drive for a few months to see how they get on' is advising that patient to break the law of the land, which is liberal enough as it is. The overall dangers of cycling are not so great, but there should be no cycling in traffic or on main roads.*

* It must be stressed that an epileptic *still having fits* should not drive, cycle, or swim. The remarks apply only to those who are under excellent control, or who have very infrequent attacks purely in their sleep.

Can I play games and swim? Normal games can be played. If swimming is always in the close company of someone who knows the history, it seems reasonable to permit this.* Rock climbing, rope climbing in the gym, etc. are obviously unwise.

What about getting married? There is nothing against an epileptic getting married for the patient should aim to live a normal social and domestic life, but their future spouse must, of course, know about the epilepsy.

Can I never have any children? Of course you can have children. An epileptic's child has a fractionally greater chance of having epilepsy than a non-epileptic's child, but it is only fractionally greater. If an epileptic marries another epileptic the chances increase considerably and such risks should probably be discouraged.

Cerebral and Spinal Tumours

Will I be cured by this operation? Each case being different, the nurse should make sure what the surgeon would wish her to say. If it is certain that the tumour is benign (see list on p. 86) the answer would be that the tumour can be cured completely. Be wary, however, of promising complete recovery of an existing disability such as impaired vision, or a paralysed limb. These are likely to return to normal, but they may not.

If the tumour is malignant, the aim of the operation is to improve matters as much as possible, and the patient should be told not to be concerned if symptoms are a little worse for a few days afterwards. The relatives should be told exactly what the situation and likely outlook are. If the surgeons and physicians in charge of the patient make the practice of giving deep X-ray treatment to malignant cerebral tumours, the patient and relatives should be warned before the operation that this might be necessary, but the wisdom of this form of therapy is debatable in many cases.

Disseminated Sclerosis

Will I become bedridden? This may be so, but what is there to be gained by depriving patients of all hope? The facts are that some people have a few relapses and then no further trouble; others have relapses and remissions throughout life, but never become disabled; others do have a slowly increasing disability, but never serious enough for them to lose their jobs. Only a proportion rapidly advance to total and pitiful incapacity, and in the early stages it is kinder to concentrate on the brighter prospects, for though the

* See footnote on previous page.

patient who becomes bedridden may think you made a mistake, you will have given him several years of hope and freedom from anxiety.

Will these symptoms develop again? They may do, but not necessarily, and there may be many years interval.

Is there no treatment? So far nothing is known which will prevent relapses, wild claims are not justified, and patients must be warned against spending large sums of money on worthless 'cures'. Something can be done, however, in acute relapses in early cases (see p. 103). Complex diets are of quite unproven value.

What about marriage and children? There is nothing to stop marriage, and no danger of passing the disease on. (This may not be 100% true, but it is almost so.) Pregnancy may be followed by a relapse, but the subsequent remission may be prolonged, and there need not finally be much greater disability. It is wise, however, to limit the family. The more relapses there are, the more permanent damage there may be; and the more young children there are, the more difficult it is for a partly disabled mother to cope with them.

Cerebrovascular Accidents

Is this likely to happen again? In all types of vascular accidents this is the main question. An honest answer is that this is a possibility. It is important that if there are any measures available to lessen the risk, these should be taken. In cerebral thrombosis, the main hope of prevention is if it is shown that the lesion lies in the carotid artery. In cerebral haemorrhage, the hypertension requires treatment. In subarachnoid haemorrhage, if the aneurysm is found and successfully clipped then one can say that the danger is over.

What can I do to prevent it? Carry out the treatment your doctor orders regularly. Apart from this there is little evidence that any particular thing influences the danger of recurrence.

Cerebral Trauma

Will my sense of smell return? If there has been a true traumatic anosmia, lasting several weeks, it will not.

How soon should I go back to work? As soon as possible; within a month if the physical condition otherwise permits. The longer away from work, the harder it is to get back to it.

Is there a danger of fits developing? Unless there has been a depressed fracture with penetration of the meninges, the danger is remote. A fit immediately after the injury need not mean that others will follow. After very severe cerebral laceration the chances are about 45%.

Might I get into the same state as the man next door who has been a nervous wreck since his accident, etc., etc.? If this question is asked following a relatively mild injury, the answer is that, providing work is resumed within a few weeks and claims for compensation are not involved, there is no such danger. In cases of grave injury with prolonged coma, there may be permanent dementia, but these are not the patients who ask the question.

General Questions

Can I go on the Continent for my holiday? Yes, certainly, but if the disease requires regular treatment, make sure supplies will be sufficient.

Can I travel by air? Modern aircraft are a lot less liable to cause further damage to any neurological lesion than a bumpy ride in an ambulance!

Will I be able to emigrate to Canada/Australia? Many places require a certificate of 'cure' if there has been any neurological disease. This, therefore, prohibits most patients with conditions such as disseminated sclerosis and epilepsy, but if there has been freedom from fits for many years, some countries allow admission.

Why has this happened to me? I have always led a good life. There is often a feeling that sexual misbehaviour and alcoholic excess must account for mysterious disease. Apart from neurosyphilis or chronic alcoholism there is no relationship whatsoever, and it is wiser to admit ignorance as to why certain people have certain things. If you get involved in trying to find an explanation, you will regret it.

APPENDIX

Throughout the appendix tables S.I. units are used with old values given in brackets.

URINE ANALYSIS IN NEUROLOGICAL DISEASE

	Abnormality	Associated diseases
Albumen	Present++	Renal disease with coma, fits; collagen disease
Sugar	Present	Diabetes with coma, neuritis, after subarachnoid haemorrhage
Casts; red cells	Present	As for albumen
Amino-acids	Excess	Wilson's disease Other rare metabolic diseases
Copper	Excess	Wilson's disease
Porphyrins	Excess porphyrins Porphobilinogen present	Polyneuritis with mental changes
Creatine and Creatinine	Excess	Muscular dystrophies
Hormones	Excess 17-hydroxy-corticosteroids	Cushings disease
	Very low ketosteroids	Hypopituitarism
Barbiturates (or other drugs)	Excess	Coma from overdosage

FAECAL ANALYSIS IN NEUROLOGICAL DISEASE

	Abnormality	Associated diseases
Occult Blood	Present	Search for primary growth in suspected neurological metastases
Fat	Excess	Polyneuropathy with steatorrhoea
Parasites	Ova present	Fits; encephalitis
Viruses	Present	Various virus diseases, especially poliomyelitis and other lymphocytic meningitis

C.S.F. ANALYSIS

Some changes may be found in the C.S.F. in almost any neurological disease; this table illustrates those which are of greatest diagnostic value.

	Normal	Type of abnormality	Associated.diseases
Cells	Less than 5×10^6 per litre (5 per cu mm)	High polymorph count	Bacterial meningitis
	No polymorphs	High lymphocyte count	Viral meningitis Poliomyelitis Encephalitis Tuberculous meningitis
		Raised lymphocyte count	As above but also— Disseminated sclerosis Metastases Collagen diseases
		Mixed count	Early viral infections Early tuberculous meningitis Neurosyphilis
		Red blood cells plus xanthochromia	Subarachnoid haemorrhage
Protein	0·15–0·45 g per litre (15–45 mg per 100 ml)	Raised 0·5–1 g (50–100 mg)	Too many diseases to have diagnostic value
		Very high: 1·5 g+ (150 mg+)	Infective Polyneuritis Neurofibromas Below spinal block
Gamma globulin	Less than 10% of total protein	Above 20%	Disseminated sclerosis Neurosyphilis
IgG		Raised	Collagen diseases
Sugar	3·5–4·5 mmol per litre (60–80 mg per 100 ml)	High	Diabetes
		Low <2 mmol (<40 mg)	Bacterial meningitis Tuberculous meningitis Carcinomatosis of the meninges
Chlorides	120–130 mmol per litre (720–750 mg per 100 ml)	Low <111 mmol (<650 mg)	Tuberculous meningitis
Lange curve	0000000000 (a few 1's may be present)	5544321000 (paretic)	General paralysis of the insane (W.R. ++) Disseminated sclerosis (W.R. −) Some viral infections
Progressively smaller amounts of C.S.F. are added to 10 tubes of colloidal gold solution. The colours produced are given numbers from 5–0.		0145432100 (luetic)	Tabes dorsalis

BLOOD ANALYSIS IN NEUROLOGICAL DISEASE

	Type of abnormality	Associated diseases
Red cell count 4–5 × 10^{12} per litre (4–5 million per cu mm)	Macrocytic anaemia (pernicious anaemia)	Subacute combined degeneration
White cell count 6–10 × 10^{9} per litre (6–10 thous. per cu mm)	Leucocytosis	Cerebral or spinal bacterial infections
	Glandular fever cells Leukaemia	Polyneuritis Cerebral deposits; peripheral nerve lesions
Sedimentation Rate < 10 mm in 1 hour	High 20–100	Metastases Infections
	Very high 100+	Collagen diseases Myeloma
Blood Sugar **4–10 mmol per litre** **(70–180 mg per 100 ml)** **random**	**High > 11 mmol** **(> 200 mg)**	**Diabetic coma; neuritis**
3–5 mmol per litre **(50–90 mg per 100 ml)** **fasting**	**Low < 2 mmol** **(< 40 mg)**	**Hypoglycaemic coma; fits**
Blood Urea **3·5–6·5 mmol per litre** **(20–40 mg per 100 ml)**	**High > 14 mmol** **(> 100 mg)**	**Uraemic coma; fits**
Serum Calcium **± 2·5 mmol per litre** **(± 10 mg)**	**Low < 2 mmol** **(< 8 mg)**	**Tetany**
Serum potassium **3·5–5·5 mmol per litre** **(3·5–5·5 mEq per litre)**	**Low < 3·5 mmol** **(< 3·5 mEq)**	**Flaccid paralysis**
Serum proteins **Alb. 30–50 g per litre (3–5 per 100 ml)** **Glob. 20–35 g per litre (2–3·5 g per 100 ml)**	**Reversed albumen/globulin ratio**	**Collagen diseases** **Myeloma**
Serum B.12 150–900 ng per litre (150–900 µµg per ml)	Very low < 100 ng (< 100 µµg)	Subacute combined degeneration
Serum folate > 3 µg per litre (> 3 mµg per ml)	Low < 2 µg (< 2 mµg)	Some dementias Anticonvulsant toxicity

BLOOD ANALYSIS—Continued

	Type of abnormality	Associated diseases
Serum acid phosphatase <8 I.U. per litre (<5 K.A. units)	High >10 I.U. (>6 K.A. units)	Secondaries from prostatic carcinoma
Serum alkaline phosphatase 20—100 I.U. per litre (3–14 K.A. units)	High >120 I.U. (>20 K.A.)	Paget's disease
Serum pyruvate <100 μmol (<1 mg)	High >100 μmol (>1 mg)	Vit. B.1. deficiency
Serum copper 11–22 μmol per litre (70–140 μg per 100 ml)	Low <8 μmol (<50 μg)	Wilson's disease
Serum creatine phosphokinase*	High	Muscular dystrophy Myositis
Agglutinations	Diagnostic levels	Various viral and leptospiral diseases

* Figures depend on methods used

INDEX